AF698392

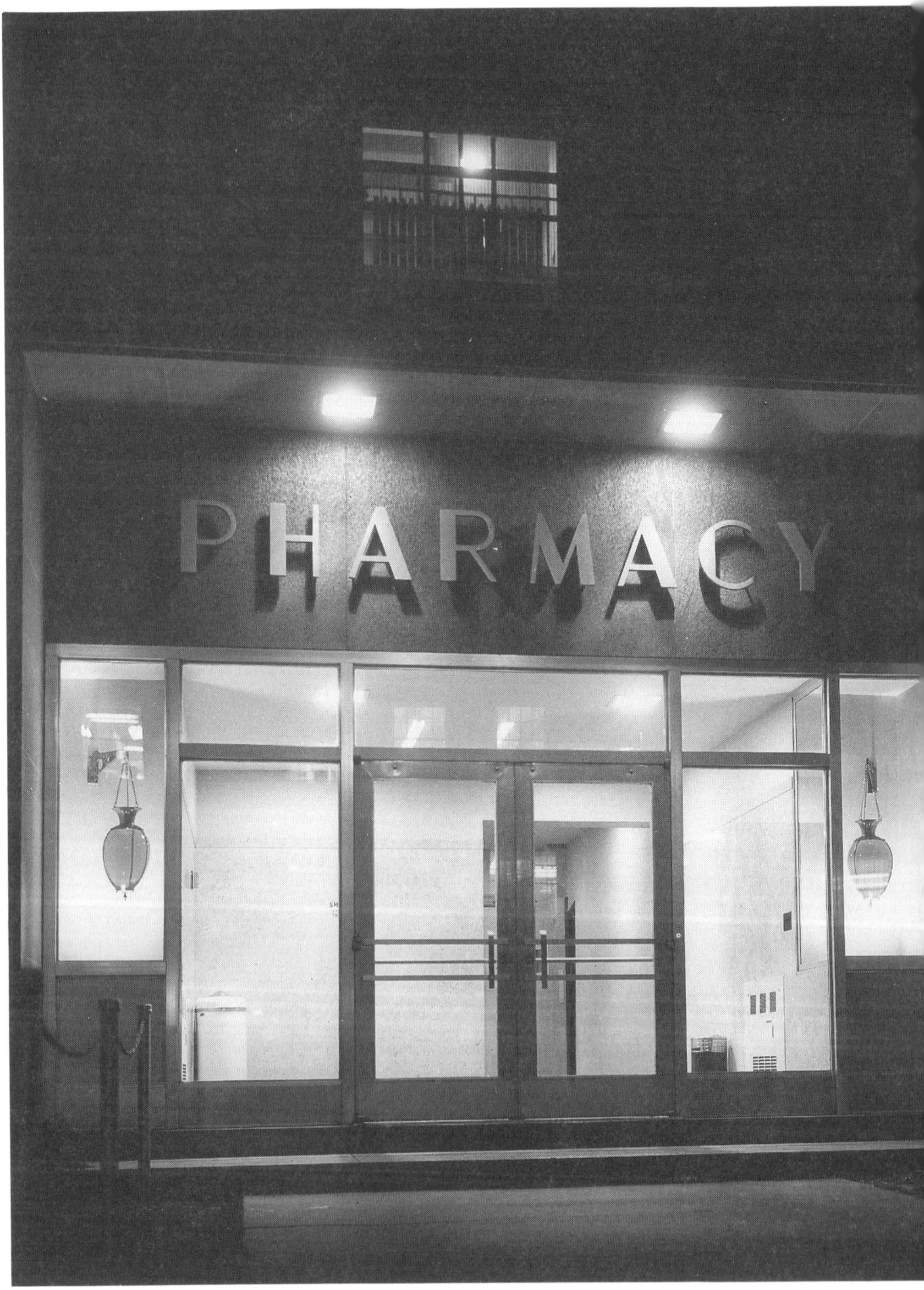
PHARMACY

THE UNIVERSITY OF WISCONSIN

SCHOOL OF PHARMACY

Its First Century

BY

CARL BUCKNER

KENNETH A. CONNORS

JOHN PARASCANDOLA

GLENN SONNEDECKER

GEORGE ZOGRAFI

Office of University Publications
Madison, Wisconsin, 1997

In Commemoration:
The Sesquicentennial of the University of Wisconsin
• Chartered by the State Constitution and Law of 1848 •

General Editor
Glenn Sonnedecker

Publication supported in part by a grant from
THE STATE HISTORICAL SOCIETY OF WISCONSIN
Albert H. Hollister Fund

ISBN 0-9658834-0-X
LC CCN 97-20473 For LC CIP data, see page 240

©1997 by The Board of Regents of the University of Wisconsin System.
All rights reserved. Printed in the United States of America
Distributor:
School of Pharmacy, University of Wisconsin–Madison
Madison, Wisconsin, 53706

Table of Contents

Appendices

Foreword

WHETHER education shapes practice more than practice shapes education can be debated. Beyond question is that the Midwestern state universities have been an important professionalizing force in occupations that are based on science. Pharmacy illustrates this point year in and year out, through the service of UW alumni to Wisconsin citizens. At this writing, the five different degrees available through the School of Pharmacy stand among 149 baccalaureate programs, 172 master's programs, and 125 doctorate and professional programs. How dramatic the contrast with 1883 when the newborn pharmacy program stood at UW–Madison among only 10 "courses" (curricula) listed in the University's *Catalogue*. This contrast suggests the remarkable development that the University's sesquicentennial observance celebrates. Pharmacy has both benefited by and contributed to the fifteen decades of educational endeavor; so it seems particularly appropriate, to help commemorate the anniversary, that the School add this small volume to the University's historical record.

The chapters of this book present the history of pharmacy at the University of Wisconsin and how it has advanced since 1883. The rapid pace of an ever changing society and the continual alterations in pharmacy practice and education resulting from modern technology present a challenge to the profession. The challenge is even greater to pharmacy educators in their efforts to train health professionals for the future.

The authors have filled a niche in the historical literature about the health sciences in Wisconsin, and thereby contributed also to the history of American pharmaceutical education. We appreciate that they have done that as a voluntary contribution, additional to their usual work. We likewise appreciate that the State Historical Society of Wisconsin has joined with the School of Pharmacy to make publication possible.

Melvin H. Weinswig, Ph.D.
Dean, School of Pharmacy
University of Wisconsin–Madison

Preface

OLD WAYS of creating pharmacists were challenged when American pharmacy connected with state universities during the second half of the nineteenth century. Pharmacy as a calling accorded with the openness of these heartland institutions toward educating for middle-class occupations that served practical needs of the citizenry—an orientation beyond the tradition of oldline Eastern universities. A reform of pharmaceutical education thus began, unappreciated by some practitioners. It evolved into a constructive trend nationally, in which—as these historical pages show—Wisconsin played a major role.

Over the decades, the University of Wisconsin exemplified the erratic course of this reform movement in pharmaceutical education. Enhancing, as it did, one facet of health care in the state, the School of Pharmacy merits historical examination; but no systematic account has appeared since 1900, when a historical volume, *The Badger Pharmacist*, was put together by the scientist-historian Edward Kremers and published by students of the School of Pharmacy. One of Kremers' successors as head of the School, Dean George Zografi, was motivated by the School's centennial to conceive the volume here presented and to appoint its co-authors, all of whom are or were members of the pharmacy faculty.

In carrying out that mission we have tried to create an account concise and readable, yet sufficiently documented to the sources to provide an enduring reference value. We have tried to avoid the chauvinism that can mar self-generated histories of institutions. However, with space at a premium, we may have let some foibles and failures go unnoticed.

The average reader imagined by the authors is an interested graduate. Therefore many details of interest to historians or educators have been placed in appendices or omitted altogether. If additional information is wanted, sources often can be discerned from the endnotes of each chapter. After a chapter on the founding, the book is organized around four broad themes for the sake of coherence, thus clarifying the relatedness of events—better, it seemed to us, than the alternative of a chronologic recital of the entire century. Chapter-authors understood that the scope of their assignment was the first hundred years of the School. However, they have mentioned, briefly and variably, some post–1983 events and data whose historical significance seemed apparent.

It has not been feasible to discuss all the larger issues that agitated pharmaceutical educators across the century and across the country; nor has it been feasible to peer into the minds and laboratories of numerous faculty members who gained national recognition and, in some other context, merit historical assessment. We do hope these pages paint a meaningful picture of how the UW School of Pharmacy came of age as an integral part of a major state university and contribute to an understanding of how the School served Wisconsin and the wider world of pharmaceutical endeavor.

G.S.

Acknowledgments

The creation of this volume benefitted greatly from the cooperative research and spirit among the five co-authors and from the consistent support by the Dean's office, notably by Dean Melvin H. Weinswig. Many others who contributed in ways large and small have our appreciation.

This book became possible largely because of the encouragement and generous support to publication offered by the State Historical Society of Wisconsin and by the UW School of Pharmacy. It is noteworthy that the present project is but the latest in a series of publications and archival projects in the history of pharmacy that the Historical Society has supported through a bequest by the Madison pharmacist, Albert H. Hollister (1843–1910). The School of Pharmacy itself provided a publishing subvention and a Project Assistant for a year during the historical investigations. Gregory J. Higby undertook that assignment while still a doctoral candidate. He strengthened the account in these pages by unearthing considerable historical data (including the statistics on graduates) and by searching out part of the photographs.

The co-authors are likewise grateful for the cooperation of other members of the faculty and staff of the University. We are indebted especially to Sandra and Tim Gossens, Larry Mindel, and Linda Frei for access to their School records of recent decades; to the UW Office of the Registrar, particularly Richard A. Jahnke, for student statistics from the beginning onward; to UW Librarians and Archivists, particularly the pharmacy librarian Dolores Nemec, for constant helpfulness; and to Mary Capener and staff in the School Office, especially Joni Mitchell, whose computer expertise and patience contributed immeasurably to putting the School's history between covers.

The design of the book and other publishing responsibilities have been in the competent hands of University Publications at UW–Madison, notably Linda R. Kietzer and Nancy B. Rinehart. Chapter I on "The Founding," by John Parascandola, has been preprinted in modified form in *Pharmacy in History* 38 (1996): 51–61.

The photographs here reproduced were kindly loaned by the Frederick B. Power Pharmaceutical library (KRF). Most of the illustrations were photographed for the School of Pharmacy over the decades by the UW–Extension's Photographic Media Center and its predecessors. Exceptions are the several photographs supplied by the UW–Madison Archives and by faculty members: the portrait of A.H. Hollister by the Curtiss Studio of Madison; the group photograph of representatives of the School of Pharmacy, Board of Pharmacy, and Wisconsin Pharmaceutical Association taken by the Diemer Photographic Laboratory of Madison; and photographs of student groups by Kappa Psi Fraternity. The graphs in the book were devised by Carl Buckner (for Chapter 4) and by Kenneth A. Connors (for Chapter 5).

Common Abbreviations Utilized

The following abbreviations and short titles are utilized in both the narrative and footnotes, after being spelled out in full at least once.

AACP:	American Association of Colleges of Pharmacy
AAPS:	American Association of Pharmaceutical Scientists
ACPE:	American Council on Pharmaceutical Education
ACPF:	American Conference of Pharmaceutical Faculties (predecessor of AACP)
ACS:	American Chemical Society
Announcement:	*University of Wisconsin, Announcement of Courses*
APhA:	American Pharmaceutical Association
APS:	Academy of Pharmaceutical Sciences (APhA)
Archives:	University of Wisconsin–Madison Archives
Bulletin:	*Bulletin of the University of Wisconsin, School of Pharmacy*
Catalog(ue):	*Catalogue of the University of Wisconsin*
KRF:	Edward Kremers Reference Files, in the F.B. Power Pharmaceutical Library, University of Wisconsin–Madison
n.:	Note (with author surname and number, e.g., n. 15) refers reader to an earlier footnote giving the full reference.
School:	School of Pharmacy, University of Wisconsin (used interchangeably here with the term Department)
SHSW:	State Historical Society of Wisconsin
UW, or University:	University of Wisconsin
WPhA:	Wisconsin Pharmaceutical (now: Pharmacists) Association

CHAPTER 1

The Founding

BY JOHN PARASCANDOLA

THE DECADE of the 1880s was a period of intense activity in organizing and professionalizing American pharmacy. Nineteen new state pharmaceutical associations were founded in this decade, equalling the number of such organizations created during the previous century in the United States. Pharmacy practice laws were enacted in more than twenty states and territories in the 1880s, about twice the number of laws enacted up to that time. At least sixteen schools of pharmacy were established in the period 1880 to 1889, about as many as had originated prior to 1880.[1] It was in the midst of this flurry of pharmaceutical activity that the University of Wisconsin School of Pharmacy was founded in 1883.

Pharmaceutical Education in Nineteenth-Century America

In early decades of the nation's history, the young would-be pharmacist received a pharmaceutical education by apprenticeship with a pharmacist or physician. Indeed, apprenticeship was to remain the chief or only form of professional education for a majority of American pharmacists until the twentieth century. In the absence of laws governing pharmacy (except in a few isolated locales) and of the traditional standards of the old European guilds, this apprenticeship training was extremely variable in quality and length and could hardly be called an educational system.[2]

Some efforts were made to provide more formal pharmaceutical instruction in early America. Course work in pharmacy was offered in the first American medical school, founded in Philadelphia in 1765, and in various medical schools established thereafter. This instruction was aimed not at the pharmacist, but at future medical practitioners, who often dispensed their own medicines.[3]

Perhaps the first effort by an American pharmacist to provide formal pharmaceutical instruction was made by a Philadelphia apothecary and chemist, James Cutbush, who advertised a series of lectures on the theory and practice of pharmacy in 1812. In 1816, physician James Mease received permission from the Board of Trustees of the University of Pennsylvania to use a University building for his lectures on pharmacy. Apparently both of these ventures were short lived, and the true beginnings of American pharmaceutical education awaited the establishment of the Philadelphia College of Pharmacy in 1821.[4]

Although the course of lectures by Mease was transitory, it may have influenced John Redman Coxe, professor of materia medica and dean of the medical faculty at the University of Pennsylvania. At Coxe's suggestion, the Board of Trustees resolved in 1819 that the teaching of the pharmaceutical art should be a part of the duties of the professor of materia medica and pharmacy, and that a course of lectures for intended practitioners of pharmacy should be established.

Coxe soon developed an ambitious plan for a pharmacy degree to be granted on the basis of three years of work in an apothecary shop and two courses of lectures on chemistry, materia medica and pharmacy. The pattern was similar to that required for medical students, who also had to serve a three-year apprenticeship and attend two courses of lectures, although the medical curriculum was broader in scope. Coxe recognized the need to win the support of the pharmaceutical profession, and he obtained the recommendation of sixteen prominent Philadelphia pharmacists before presenting his proposal to the Board of Trustees. The inclusion of a statement that it might be "proper to grant an honorary degree of the same nature to those apothecaries of standing in Philadelphia who may sanction the proposed plan" probably made it easier for these pharmacists to support the proposal.

On February 6, 1821, the Board of Trustees adopted Coxe's plan for awarding the "Master of Pharmacy" degree. The reaction of the druggists and apothecaries of Philadelphia was largely negative. Various objections were offered: the plan would lead to fewer apothecaries, freedom of trade would be interfered with, and the cost of education would be more than most apothecaries could afford. The question was raised as to whether members of the medical faculty were the best judges of the qualifications of apothecaries. Concern was also expressed that those apothecaries not granted an honorary degree and unable or unwilling to obtain it by examination would lose the confidence of the public.

Only four days after the plan was published, a meeting of apothecaries and druggists was held in Carpenters' Hall to discuss the matter, and at a second meeting on April 12 a committee recommended that an association of druggists and apothecaries of Philadelphia be organized and that one of its functions be to establish a school of pharmacy. Thus was born the Philadelphia College of Apothecaries—changed the following year to the Philadelphia College of Pharmacy—the first association of pharmacists in the United States. The University's pharmacy program quietly passed away, while the new independent school established by the pharmacists of Philadelphia, the first school of pharmacy in this country, survived and prospered.

Formal instruction at the Philadelphia College of Pharmacy began in November 1821 with two courses of lectures, one on materia medica and pharmacy and the other on pharmaceutical and general chemistry, both given in the evening. No degree was granted, but in 1826 it was decided that students who had served an apprenticeship, attended the course of lectures twice, and passed an examination would be designated as graduates of the College.[5]

In time pharmacists of other cities followed the lead of their Philadelphia colleagues and formed local associations, and some of these associations established educational institutions. The Massachusetts College of Pharmacy was founded in Boston in 1823, and offered occasional lectures, but apparently it did not provide regular instruction until 1867. The third association to be established, the College of Pharmacy of the City (and County) of New York, did operate a school from its founding in 1829. Two other local pharmaceutical associations were offering formal pharmacy instruction before the Civil War, the Maryland College of Pharmacy (1840) and the Chicago College of Pharmacy (1859). Only one other educational institution offered a pharmacy degree in antebellum America, the Medical College of Louisiana (later part of Tulane University), which instituted a pharmacy course in 1838, but graduated no more than one or two students a year before the 1860s.

Pharmacy education in this period was a part-time affair. Students worked in a drugstore during the day and attended lectures in the evening. Apprenticeship was still considered to be the most important part of the pharmacist's education.

The typical pharmacy program included lectures on two or three nights a week for about four or five months of the year. At first there were two courses, one in pharmaceutical chemistry and one in materia medica and pharmacy combined, but later pharmacy was split off as a separate, third course. The student was usually required to attend two courses of each of the lectures, which meant that he attended the same lectures for a second time in the following year. This procedure was also common in medical education at the time. There was no laboratory instruction, and the teachers, who were more often physicians than pharmacists in the antebellum period, did not earn their living from the fees that they earned from the courses.

It must be kept in mind that only a small percentage of those entering the pharmaceutical profession in America before the Civil War had ever attended a college of pharmacy, and an even smaller percentage were graduates of such a college. There were only 513 graduates of American pharmacy schools up through 1860, and nearly four-fifths of this group were from the Philadelphia College of Pharmacy. The number of graduates significantly increased in the latter part of the century with the founding of many new schools of pharmacy, but it was estimated as late as 1896 that only about 12 percent of the nation's pharmacists had any technical education other than practice experience. Although almost every state had enacted a pharmacy practice act (requiring passage of a licensure examination) by the end of the nineteenth century, no state required graduation from a school of pharmacy as a prerequisite to licensure until New York became the first to take that step in 1905.[6]

The pattern of part-time pharmaceutical education established by the independent schools was transformed when instruction began to be incorporated into the state universities. The Medical College of South Carolina was apparently the first state institution to produce graduates in pharmacy in 1867, but pharmaceutical education had a precarious existence there until the end of the century. It was at the University of Michigan, beginning in 1868, that bold innovations were made that significantly influenced the direction of American pharmaceutical education.

Pharmacy instruction had been offered at Michigan since 1860 as a part of the medical curriculum. In 1868, however, the University established a separate "Course of Study in Pharmacy" within the Department of Science, Literature and Arts. The course, which required one and a half to two years to complete, led to the diploma of "Pharmaceutical Chemist" (Ph.C.) for those who submitted a satisfactory thesis and successfully passed the examination. Michigan's program was characterized by a strong emphasis on basic science education, including laboratory instruction, and it essentially required the full-time attendance of students.[7]

The curriculum as described in the 1868–69 catalog of the University included: "Lectures upon Chemical Physics, Inorganic and Organic Chemistry, and Toxicology; Lectures upon Materia Medica; Recitations and Lectures upon Practical Pharmacy; thorough and systematic practice in Qualitative Chemical Analysis, optional; practice in Medico-legal Analysis of Poisons, and in Analysis of Urine; Systematic exercises in Metrology, Acidimetry, Alkalimetry, Distillation and Alcoholometry, and in the preparation of Pharmacopoeial and Chemical Compounds and Medicinal Preparations." The catalog noted that students in the pharmacy course could be admitted to classes in botany, English, German, French, Latin or any other subject for which they had adequate preparation.[8]

What the Michigan program did not include, however, was the traditional requirement of a period of apprenticeship before graduation. This omission was heretical in the eyes of the schools of pharmacy operated by associations, which still viewed the apprenticeship as the heart of the pharmacist's education. At the 1871 meeting of the American Pharmaceutical Association, Michigan's School of Pharmacy failed to win recognition as a "college of pharmacy," within the meaning of the Association's constitution and by-laws, because it was not controlled by pharmacists and did not require the "proper practical training" (i.e., apprenticeship) of its graduates.

At that meeting the head of the pharmacy course, physician-chemist Albert B. Prescott, offered a defense of the Michigan philosophy. Prescott outlined the advantages of a real scientific education, including laboratory experience, and argued that apprenticeship would be a much more meaningful learning experience for those who had already completed college work in the fundamental sciences. Since few states had pharmacy laws in 1871, however, there was no legal requirement for an apprenticeship and it is understandable that pharmacist-educators of the period felt that the colleges should accept this responsibility for their graduates. After the passage of state pharmacy laws and the establishment of licensure requirements, the responsibility for apprenticeship training was eventually shifted from the colleges to the state boards of pharmacy.[9]

For a time the University of Michigan stood alone, but eventually the concept of full-time pharmaceutical education based on laboratory science became the rule rather than the exception. As other state universities began to establish pharmacy programs in the last two decades of the nineteenth century, they adopted many of the innovations introduced at Michigan. In time, the old-line association schools had to follow suit. Until well into the twentieth century, however, there remained a marked differentiation among American schools of pharmacy of whatever type (state university, private university, association, or proprietary) in length, type and level of instruction.[10]

The University of Wisconsin Creates a Department of Pharmacy

The first state university to follow the Michigan model was the University of Wisconsin. Unlike the Michigan program, which was established without the cooperation of the pharmacists of the state (many in fact opposing the idea), the Wisconsin department of pharmacy was founded as a result of the initiative of the newly-created state pharmaceutical association.

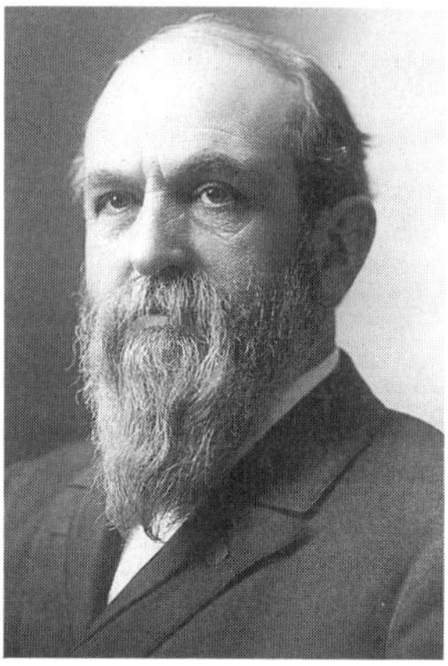

An influential advocate of establishing a department of pharmacy at the University was Albert H. Hollister, a Madison pharmacist. Other Wisconsin pharmacists especially supportive during the early years were Adam Conrath of Milwaukee, Edwin Sumner of Madison, Frederick Robinson of Kenosha, and John A. Dadd of Milwaukee.

During the last third of the nineteenth century, the pharmacists of state after state, with the encouragement of the American Pharmaceutical Association, organized state pharmaceutical associations. The first of these was established in Maine in 1867. More than half of them were established in little more than a decade, centering in the 1880s. During this same period many state pharmacy laws were enacted, and the state associations, many of which had been organized partly for the purpose of fostering such legislation, played a key role in securing the passage of these acts by state legislators.

The pharmacists of Wisconsin were no exception to this national trend towards organization in pharmacy in the late nineteenth century. Milwaukee pharmacists, led by German immigrants, successfully fought for the passage of a law to regulate the practice of pharmacy in their city in 1876, although they did not succeed in their efforts to establish a local pharmaceutical society. A Janesville pharmacist, Edward B. Heimstreet, encouraged by the General Secretary of the American Pharmaceutical Association, John M. Maisch, began the organization of Wisconsin pharmacists in 1878 by forming a local, informal group of seven pharmacists of Janesville. The following year he organized the Rock County Pharmaceutical Society. In 1880 the Society met in Madison, the state capitol, and invited pharmacists from around the state to attend the meeting for the purpose of forming a state pharmaceutical association.

The Wisconsin Pharmaceutical Association was founded at this meeting. At the first annual meeting of the state association in 1881, President John Dadd reminded the members of the importance of securing laws to regulate the practice of pharmacy. A committee was appointed to work for the passage of a pharmacy law in Wisconsin, and such legislation was enacted in 1882.[11]

When the Wisconsin Pharmaceutical Association met in 1882, President Frederick Robinson of Kenosha suggested the creation of a school of pharmacy. "By reference to the last annual report of the Board of Regents," he said, "I find that the State University already embraces a good chemical laboratory, and that its instructional force includes a chemist and a botanist. I would therefore recommend the adoption of some steps to secure the establishment of a chair of Pharmacy and Materia Medica, in connection with the University, in order that the druggists of the State may be supplied with educational advantages commensurate with those offered in other branches and equal to those of any other State."[12]

In response to President Robinson's suggestion, a committee, consisting of Adam Conrath of Milwaukee, Frederick F. Prentice of Janesville, and Albert H. Hollister of Madison, was appointed to confer with the Board of Regents of the University.[13] On January 16, 1883, the Committee appeared before the Board of Regents and advocated the establishment of a Chair of Pharmacy and Materia Medica. After discussing the question, the Regents passed a resolution requesting the faculty to establish a department of instruction in Pharmacy and Materia Medica, "acceptable to the State Board, and Association of Pharmacy," which should be opened for students as soon as sufficient revenues were obtained for the appointment of a qualified professor in the subject. To resolve this financial matter, the Regents instructed their Executive Committee to ask the state legislature to increase the annual tax levy for the University.[14]

Efforts were also underway at the time to establish an agricultural experiment station at the University, and this request was combined with the request for a pharmacy chair into a single bill. The bill, which was introduced by Representative Robert J. McBride of Neillsville, increased the state tax from one-tenth to one-eighth of a mill on the dollar for the assessed valuation of taxable property and stipulated that the increase was to be used for the establishment of a chair of pharmacy and an agricultural experiment station. It was passed by the legislature in March and signed into law by the governor on April 2, 1883.[15]

Frederick Belding Power Appointed To Head Wisconsin Program

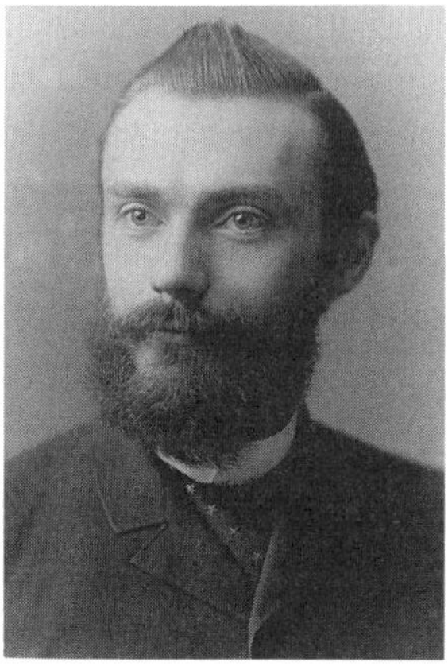

Frederick Belding Power (1853–1927), a pharmacist who earned a Ph.D. at Strassburg, became the founding director of UW's department of pharmacy at age 30. His later career made Power one of the best-known phytochemists of his time.

With the money appropriated, the task of finding a suitable occupant for the new pharmacy chair fell to the University President, John Bascom. For advice, Bascom turned to a former colleague, Ira Remsen, one of America's most prominent chemists. Remsen was acquainted with a young professor at the Philadelphia College of Pharmacy whose abilities had obviously impressed him, and he recommended the pharmacist Frederick B. Power for the position.[16]

Power was well qualified for the Wisconsin professorship of pharmacy and materia medica. He had graduated from the Philadelphia College of Pharmacy in 1874 and had worked for several years in the establishment of the noted Philadelphia pharmacist, Edward Parrish. Power had then gone to Germany to pursue further chemical and pharmaceutical studies at the University of Strassburg, where he received a Doctor of Philosophy degree in 1880 for his thesis in plant chemistry under the direction of the eminent pharmacognosist Friedrich A. Flückiger. Upon returning to the United States, Power was appointed professor of analytical chemistry at the Philadelphia College of Pharmacy, the position that he held when called to Wisconsin. (On Power, see also p. 169.)

At its meeting on June 19, 1883, the Board of Regents approved, upon recommendation of President Bascom, the establishment of a department and professorship of pharmacy, and appointed Frederick B. Power to the position at a salary of $2,000. The state association's Committee on the School of Pharmacy was again present at this meeting, and discussed with the Board and the President questions concerning the terms for admission, the course of study, and the degree to be granted. It was decided that these matters should be referred to the newly-appointed professor of pharmacy, to be worked out by him in conjunction with the President and the state association's Committee and then brought to the Executive Committee of the Board for approval.[17]

When Power arrived in August 1883, Madison was a city with a population of somewhat more than 10,000.[18] It has been described as resembling at the time "an overgrown New England college village."[19] The University of Wisconsin, which had not yet really begun the transition from a college into a major university, was situated on a hill on the shores of Lake Mendota. Efforts had been made to establish a university even in territorial days, and when Wisconsin became a state in 1848 provision was made in the constitution for a state university. The first classes were held in February, 1849, and the first building, North Hall, was completed in 1851.[20]

By the 1880s, the main buildings on the campus were North Hall, South Hall, Main Hall (now Bascom Hall), Science Hall, Library Hall (now Music Hall), and the Washburn Observatory. All of these buildings are still standing except for Science Hall, which was destroyed by fire in 1884 (and was replaced by the present Science Hall in 1887). There were only about 400 students enrolled at the University in 1883, most of them from middle-class Wisconsin homes.[21] The student body of the early 1880s was probably similar in character to the graduating class of 1877 described below:

"All were American-born, twenty-one being natives of Wisconsin and one each of Michigan, New York, Vermont, New Hampshire, Maine, Ohio, Connecticut, Massachusetts and Illinois. Nine belonged to secret societies. Five had followed the ancient classical course, two the modern classical, and eighteen the general science; six were civil engineers and one a student of mining and metallurgy. Twenty-one were Republicans, five were Democrats, and five were neutral in politics. Six confessed to occasional use of alcohol and five to the use of tobacco; the rest asserted that they were strictly temperate. Religious affiliations were dispersed; The Congregationalists numbered three; the Presbyterians, Baptists, and Unitarians each two; one was a Roman Catholic, and one an Episcopalian. The rest disclaimed any denominational preferences."[22]

The faculty that Power joined numbered about thirty-five. His salary of $2,000 was standard for a full professor at Wisconsin at the time, only the Director of the Observatory ($3,000) and the President ($3,500) earning more. The total estimated budget of expenditures for the University in 1883–84 was only about $93,000, of which about $57,000 was earmarked for salaries.[23]

The newly-created pharmacy program was affiliated with the College of Arts, one of only three colleges at the University of Wisconsin at the time (the other two being Letters and Law). The other scientific and technical courses (such as agriculture and engineering) were also administered under the umbrella of the College of Arts in this period. The University was still small enough, however, that its internal management was apparently conducted largely by the entire faculty.[24]

Organization of the Pharmacy Program

Power arrived on the campus during summer vacation in August, while President Bascom was out of town. No arrangements had yet been made concerning the requirements of the program or the rooms that it would occupy, and instruction was scheduled to begin at the opening of the University year in early September. Not surprisingly, Power confessed to feeling "considerable perplexity and anxiety" about the situation.[25]

Power soon made the acquaintance, however, of pharmacists A. H. Hollister and Adam Conrath, both members of the State Board of Pharmacy, and of various members of the faculty. When Bascom returned to Madison, it was decided that space for the pharmacy course could be provided in South Hall, originally built as a dormitory. We are fortunate in having Power's own description of the original physical facilities of the School of Pharmacy:

"Upon the return of the President it was decided that the only rooms then available for my use were those in the first floor and south side of the building, known as South Hall. These comprised a series of apartments which had previously served as bedrooms for the students, and they were exceedingly bare and uninviting in appearance. With the aid of the university carpenter the doors were removed which had separated the two larger ones, probably the *drawing rooms*, and this space, small and narrow, after being provided with a table, gas and water, was used during the first winter as a pharmaceutical laboratory. The other smaller rooms adjoining were obliged to serve respectively as office, balance room, store rooms, etc. There was a wood stove in the laboratory, but the other rooms were not heated, and with a temperature outside of frequently 10 to 20 degrees below zero the quarters of the Professor of Pharmacy can not be said to have been particularly comfortable nor possessing 'all the modern improvements.' Through the kindness of the Professor of Botany I was permitted to use his lecture room, although this was provided with neither gas nor water. Some few experiments could be shown with the aid of an alcohol lamp, but all test-tubes or other apparatus which required cleaning had to be taken to the basement, where there was the luxury of a sink, and this work had to be done by myself."[26]

Power had much to do to keep him busy while awaiting the return of the President from vacation. He had to compile a list of the equipment and materials that he would need, to begin preparing his own lectures, to develop an announcement of the course to circulate to pharmacists of the state, and to draw up a plan for the curriculum. One of the most important and pressing tasks he faced was to make arrangements with appro-

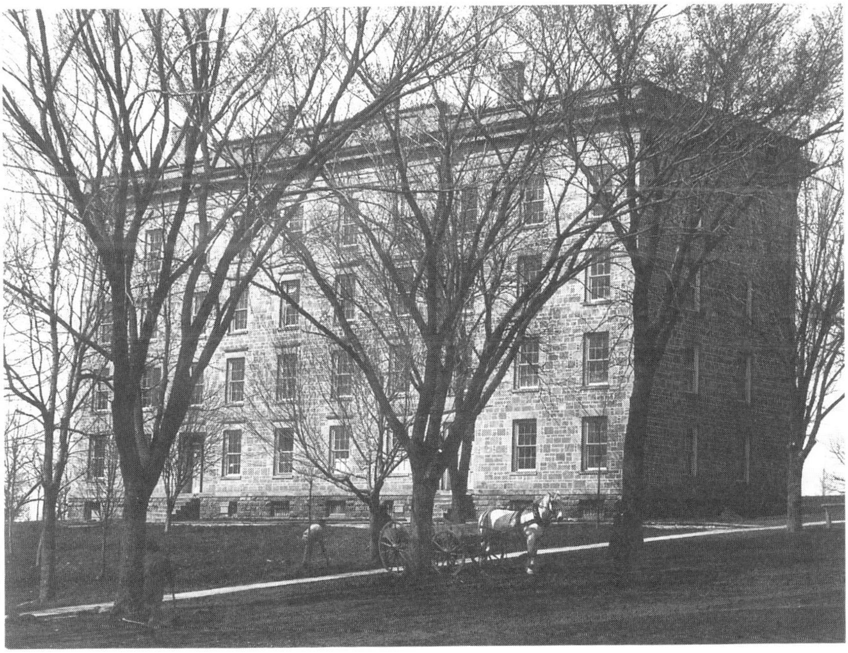

South Hall on the brow of Bascom Hill, the second building constructed on the campus, as it looked when the department of pharmacy was established there in 1883 (South side, first floor). The department's first director found that the rooms assigned to pharmacy were "exceedingly bare and uninviting."

priate members of the faculty to provide the needed instruction.

Power himself was to teach pharmacy and materia medica, but it was necessary to have the cooperation of faculty members in other disciplines, such as chemistry and botany. The first announcement of the new School included in its list of faculty (in addition to Power) William W. Daniells, John E. Davies, Charles R. Van Hise and William Trelease.[27]

Daniells (1840–1911), who was professor of chemistry, had come to Wisconsin in 1868 as professor of agriculture. The son of a Michigan farmer, he obtained a B.Sc. in 1864 and an M.S. in 1867 from the Michigan Agricultural College (later Michigan State University). In between he had studied chemistry for over a year at the Lawrence Scientific School of Harvard University. Daniells' interest at Wisconsin developed along chemical lines, and in 1880 he was made professor of chemistry, having already added teaching duties in chemistry to his responsibilities some years earlier. He was to remain on the Wisconsin faculty until his retirement in 1907. Daniells also served the state at various times as chemist to the State Geological Society, as a member of the Wisconsin State Board of Health, and as state analyst.[28]

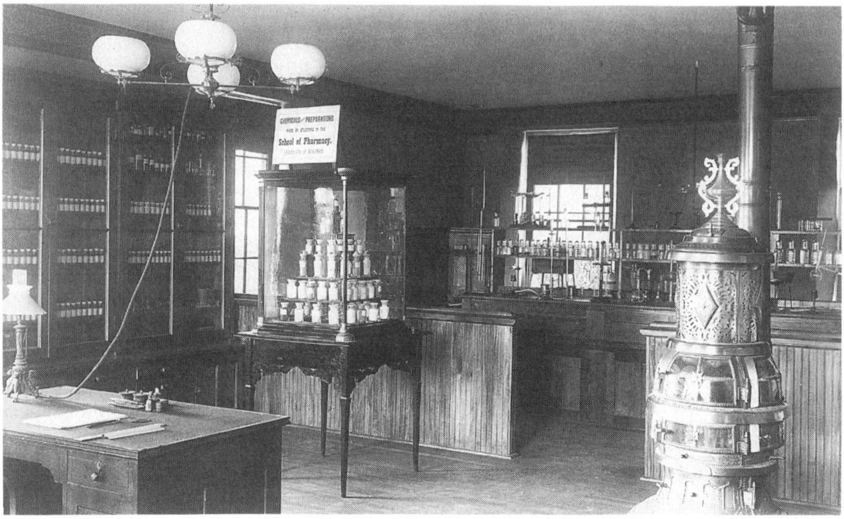

The year after the founding the department of pharmacy moved to far better quarters, occupying the entire 4th floor of South Hall. The spacious office and private laboratory of Frederick B. Power, the first Professor of Pharmacy and Materia Medica, is shown here as it looked in 1890.

The other faculty member involved in chemical instruction, Van Hise (1857–1918), was a young assistant professor of metallurgy in 1883. He obtained his B.Sc. at Wisconsin in 1880 and then served as an instructor in metallurgy while working towards his M.S., which he earned for work in geology in 1882. Although primarily interested in geology, a field to which he made significant scientific contributions, Van Hise was to teach the qualitative chemical analysis course for pharmacy students until 1886. Promoted to full professor in 1886, he went on to receive, in 1892, the first earned Ph.D. to be granted by the University of Wisconsin. A decade later, in 1903, he became President of the University, a post he held until his death in 1918.[29]

The professor of botany, Trelease (1857–1945), came to Wisconsin in 1881, after receiving his B.Sc. from Cornell in 1880 and devoting a year to post-graduate study at Harvard (from which he was eventually to earn the D.Sc. degree in 1884). In addition to his research and teaching in botany, Trelease offered what may have been the first course in bacteriology to be taught in this country. He was to leave Wisconsin in 1885 to pursue a distinguished career as director of the Missouri Botanical Garden and later as head of the Department of Botany at the University of Illinois.[30]

The connection of Davies (1839–1900), the professor of physics, with the School of Pharmacy was peripheral and tenuous. Davies graduated from Lawrence University, and received his M.D. from the Chicago Medical College in 1868, just before joining the Wisconsin faculty, of which he was to remain a member until his death.[31] His name did not appear on the faculty listing of the School of Pharmacy, however, in any annual announcement after the first one. A course in physics was listed in the first-year pharmacy curriculum in the 1883–84 University Catalog, but the evidence indicates that it was not actually given. Later catalogs no longer listed a separate course in physics. Apparently some attention was devoted to "chemical physics" (or physical chemistry) in Daniells' general chemistry course, but there is no evidence that Davies was involved in such instruction.[32]

The Regents had left the matter of deciding upon the admission requirements, the course of study, and the degree to be awarded in the hands of the professor of pharmacy, subject to the final approval of the Board's Executive Committee. These decisions were to be made in conjunction with the state association's Committee on the School of Pharmacy and the President of the University. The reports of the Committee do not mention any formal meeting with Power in this connection, but it is likely that he at least discussed his general plans with Hollister and Conrath, whom he met soon after his arrival in Madison. Power had little time to complete his plans for the pharmacy program because the University's fall term was scheduled to begin on September 5.[33]

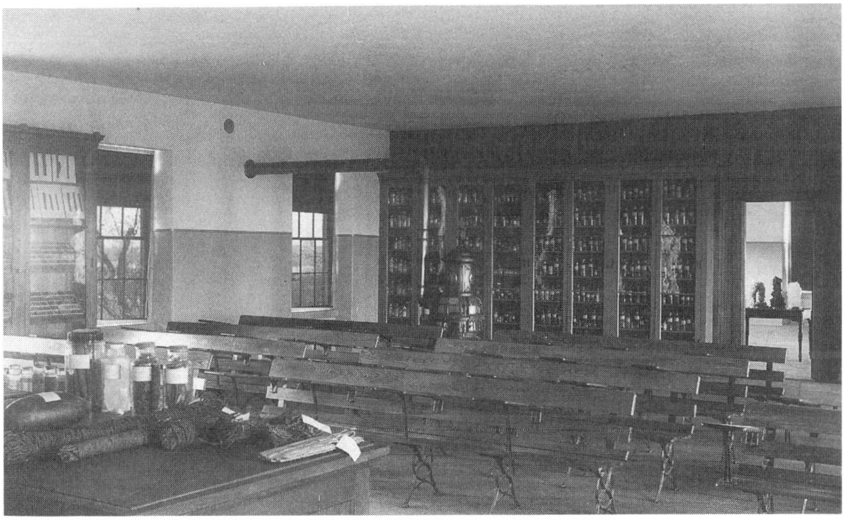

Lecture room for materia medica and pharmacy as it looked in 1890. The pot-bellied stove usually kept pharmacy students from freezing.

Program Content and Requirements

The program that Power developed was influenced both by his experience at his alma mater, the Philadelphia College of Pharmacy, and by the model established by the University of Michigan School of Pharmacy. Power's task was to develop a pharmacy course within a state university setting, and it is not surprising that he should look to Michigan, which provided the only real example of such a university-based course. On his way out to Madison, Power stopped in Ann Arbor to confer with Albert Prescott, and received from him "much encouragement and valuable suggestions regarding the organization of the school.[34] It is also likely that Power's training in Germany helped shape his thinking about pharmaceutical education, certainly at least with respect to his recognition of the importance of research in a university-based school of pharmacy.

The Wisconsin program was two years in length, as were the pharmacy courses at Michigan and the association schools, and led to the customary diploma of Graduate in Pharmacy (Ph.G.). The course did not run for the full three terms that comprised the University's academic year at the time, but occupied only the fall and winter terms, from about early September through late March (although in the first year the School was not ready to begin instruction until October l). For comparison, note that in 1883 the academic year at the Philadelphia College of Pharmacy ran from October 1 through the end of February, and at Michigan from about the beginning of October through mid to late June.[35]

Students who could provide a certificate attesting to two years of work in a pharmacy, "under the guidance of a reputable and competent preceptor," and who also showed evidence of a "good preliminary education" were admitted to the school without examination. Those failing to meet these criteria were required to take an examination covering a variety of academic subjects. By the second announcement of the pharmacy program, for the 1884–85 academic year, "a satisfactory preliminary education" had been defined as "a diploma of graduation from some standard high school, or a certificate of good standing and scholarship in a corresponding higher educational institution." Any student not meeting one of these criteria had to take an entrance examination, and no mention was made in this announcement of work experience in a pharmacy. It should be noted here that it was common at the time for students to be admitted to American schools of pharmacy without the benefit of a high school education. Provision was made to admit directly into the second (senior) year of the Wisconsin course any student who had satisfactorily completed the studies covered in the first (junior) year at another college of pharmacy.[36]

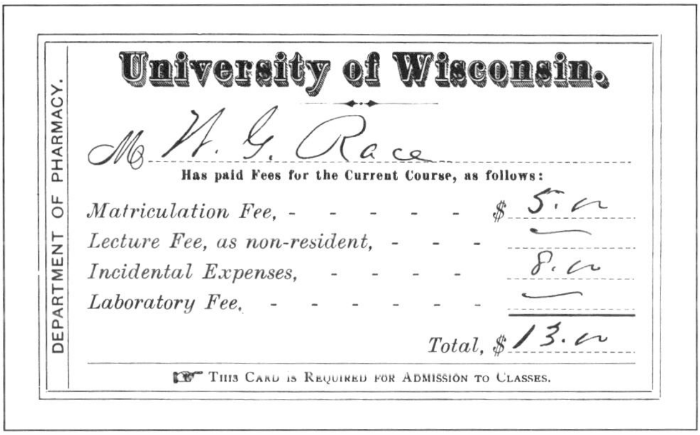
University of Wisconsin.

DEPARTMENT OF PHARMACY.

Mr. H. G. Race

Has paid Fees for the Current Course, as follows:

Matriculation Fee,	$ 5.00
Lecture Fee, as non-resident,	—
Incidental Expenses,	8.00
Laboratory Fee,	—
Total,	$ 13.00

☞ This Card is Required for Admission to Classes.

The fee card is for the fall term only a year after the University opened its department of pharmacy. Tuition has had to be increased somewhat since this receipt for $13 was issued.

The program at Wisconsin, like the one at Michigan, was intended to be full time. Lectures were not given in the evening, as they were at the association schools, and a significant amount of laboratory work was required. The required curriculum was as follows:

First Year

Practical Pharmacy and Pharmaceutical Chemistry (Power)
General Chemistry (Daniells)
Qualitative Chemical Analysis (Van Hise)
Botany (Trelease)

Second Year

Materia Medica (Pharmacognosy) (Power)
Organic Chemistry (Daniells)
Quantitative Chemical Analysis (Daniells)
Pharmaceutical Laboratory (Power)

In addition, a course in physiology (taught by the professor of Zoology, Edwin A. Birge) was listed in the second announcement of the School (1884) as being "earnestly recommended" (but not required) for all students.[37] The basic subjects covered—pharmacy, chemistry and botany—formed the backbone of every pharmacy curriculum at the time. The curriculum did not differ greatly in scope and structure from the contemporary programs at Ann Arbor or Philadelphia, although it was not quite as

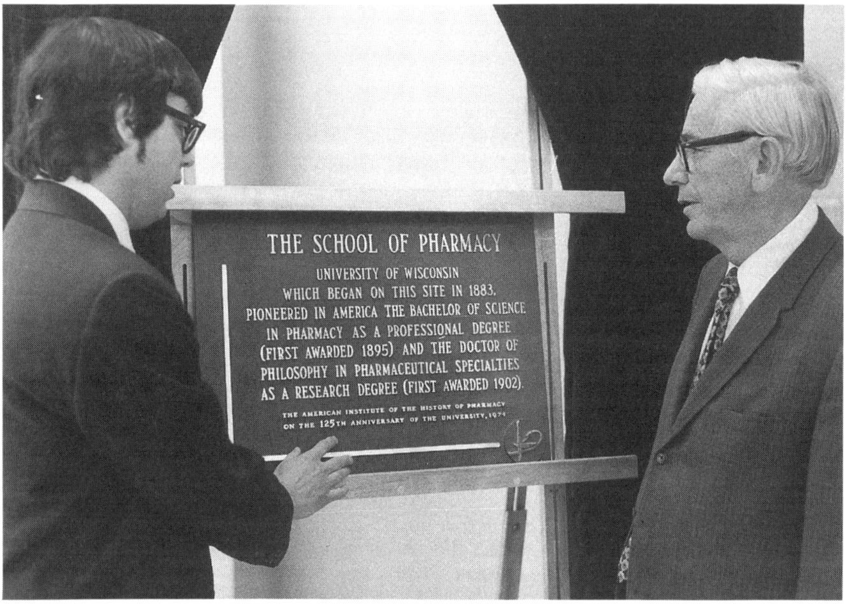
THE SCHOOL OF PHARMACY
UNIVERSITY OF WISCONSIN
WHICH BEGAN ON THIS SITE IN 1883.
PIONEERED IN AMERICA THE BACHELOR OF SCIENCE
IN PHARMACY AS A PROFESSIONAL DEGREE
(FIRST AWARDED 1895) AND THE DOCTOR OF
PHILOSOPHY IN PHARMACEUTICAL SPECIALTIES
AS A RESEARCH DEGREE (FIRST AWARDED 1902).
THE AMERICAN INSTITUTE OF THE HISTORY OF PHARMACY
ON THE 125TH ANNIVERSARY OF THE UNIVERSITY, 1974

This bronze marker on South Hall commemorates the national influence and innovative role of the UW School in American pharmaceutical education. The plaque is here being inspected at the dedication in 1974 by UW President Edwin Young (right) and the Director of the American Institute of the History of Pharmacy, John Parascandola.

encompassing as the former (which included, for example, a course in toxicology) and was more demanding than the latter (particularly with regard to laboratory work).[38]

All of the above-mentioned first-year courses were offered during the initial year of operation of the School (1883–1884), but it was not until the following year that the senior-year program was offered in its entirety. Power found it impractical, for example, to offer lectures in materia media in 1883–1884 because his specimens for demonstration had not yet arrived and because there were only a few students enrolled in the senior year (all of whom were, of course, "transfer" students). Nevertheless, three students were able to obtain their Ph. G. diploma at the end of the academic year.[39]

Unlike the University of Michigan, Wisconsin's pharmacy program included a requirement of four years of practical experience in a dispensing pharmacy for graduation. Here Power remained faithful to the tradition of the association schools in assuming responsibility for insuring that graduates received suitable apprenticeship training. This is not surprising in light of his own background and the close ties of Wisconsin's school with the pharmacists of the state.

These ties are further reflected in the requirement that candidates for the degree had to pass an examination in practical pharmacy administered by a committee composed of three members of the Wisconsin Pharmaceutical Association, in addition to an examination by the faculty on coursework. To graduate, a student also had to prepare an original essay or thesis on some subject in pharmacy, chemistry, materia medica, botany or a related science. Although this latter requirement was probably influenced by Power's commitment to scholarly research, it was not a novel idea. Both the University of Michigan School of Pharmacy and the Philadelphia College of Pharmacy, for example, were requiring a thesis for graduation in 1883.[40]

Once Power had established the requirements of the program and made arrangements for the teaching of the courses, he was able to prepare an announcement of the program for distribution to prospective students. In late August the state association mailed a copy of the first annual announcement of the School to every pharmacist in Wisconsin. The program was also publicized through notices in the pharmaceutical press.[41]

Preparations could not be completed in time to begin the pharmacy course when the University's year began on September 5, so the opening date was postponed about one month. On October 1, 1883, the *Wisconsin State Journal* reported that the "recently established pharmaceutical department of the university was opened to-day," and the first lectures were held on the following day.[42] Twenty-eight students (three or four seniors and the rest juniors) enrolled.[43] The University of Wisconsin's School of Pharmacy had been launched.

Notes and References

1. Glenn Sonnedecker, rev., *Kremers and Urdang's History of Pharmacy* (4th ed., Philadelphia, 1976), 379–386; Glenn Sonnedecker, "American Pharmaceutical Education before 1900" (Ph.D. diss., University of Wisconsin, Madison, 1952), 113.
2. Sonnedecker, "Education," (n. 1), 19–29; Glenn Sonnedecker, "Teaching Pharmacy in 19th Century America—Some Aims and Issues," *Amer. J. Pharm. Educ.*, 35(1971):381–382.
3. David Cowen, "Pharmacy in the Curriculum of American Medical Schools," *Pharm. Hist.*, 20 (1978):17–21.
4. Sonnedecker, "Education," (n. 1), 37–41; Sonnedecker, *History*, (n.1), 227.
5. On the establishment of the Philadelphia College of Pharmacy, see Joseph England, ed., *The First Century of the Philadelphia College of Pharmacy, 1821–1921* (Philadelphia, 1922), 43–80; Sonnedecker, *History*, (n.1), 189–192; Sonnedecker, "Education," (n. 1), 42–49.

6. The preceding discussion on the early development of pharmaceutical education in the United States is based on Sonnedecker, "Education," (n.1), especially 50–66, 282–287, 373–380, 411–412, and Sonnedecker, *History*, (n.1), 227–232,
7. Sonnedecker, *History*, (n. 1), 232–235; Glenn Sonnedecker, "Science in American Pharmaceutical Education of the 19th Century," *Amer. J. Pharm. Educ.*, 15(1951):205–209; Henry Manasse, "Innovation, Confrontation and Perseverance: Albert B. Prescott's Legacy to Pharmaceutical Education in America," *Pharm. Hist.*, 15(1973):22–28.
8. *University of Michigan Catalogue*, 1868–69, 56.
9. Sonnedecker, *History*, (n.1), 233–234; Manasse, (n. 7), 25–27.
10. Sonnedecker, "Science," (n. 7), 209–215.
11. On the founding of the Wisconsin Pharmaceutical Association and the passage of a pharmacy law, see Eunice Bonow Bardell, *Wisconsin Show Globe: The Wisconsin Pharmaceutical Association, 1880–1980* (Madison, 1983), 1–15.
12. "President Robinson's Address," *Proc. WPhA.*, 3(1882):15.
13. "Report of the Committee on Resolutions," *ibid.*, 59–60.
14. Minutes of the Board of Regents of the University of Wisconsin, MS, Jan. 16, 1883, vol. 3, pp. 387–388, University of Wisconsin Archives, Madison.
15. Merle Curti and Vernon Carstensen, *The University of Wisconsin: A History, 1848–1925* (Madison, 1949; 2 vols.) 1:318–319; *Supplement to the Revised Statutes of the State of Wisconsin, 1878, Containing the General Laws from 1879 to 1883*, compiled and annotated by A.L. Sanborn and J.R. Berryman (Chicago, 1883), 77.
16. Curti and Carstensen, (n. 15), I:247, 275; [Edward Kremers], "Dr. Power at Wisconsin," *Badger Pharmacist* (published by the Wisconsin Chapter of Rho Chi, Madison), (1936): No. 13, 2; Louise Power Heimke," Notes upon the Life and Achievements of Frederick Belding Power," 54-page transcript, in Edward Kremers Reference Files, F.B. Power Pharmaceutical Library, University of Wisconsin–Madison, pp. 8–9, filed under A2:Power, F.B.
17. Minutes, Board of Regents, June 19, 1883, vol. 3, p. 393.
18. The population of Madison as of the 1880 census was 10,324. See John L. Andriot, ed., *Population Abstract of the United States* (McLean, VA, 1980), 899.
19. [Kremers], "Power," (n. 16), 8.
20. Curti and Carstensen, (n. 15), I:37–152.
21. *Ibid.*, 364–393; [Kremers], "Power," (n. 16), 3–4; *Catalogue of the University of Wisconsin*, 1883–84, 23.
22. Curti and Carstensen, (n. 15), I:369.
23. *Catalogue... Wisconsin*, 1883–84, 7–8; Minutes, Board of Regents, June 19, 1883, vol. 3, pp. 399–400.
24. *Catalogue... Wisconsin*, 1887–88, 37–38; Curti and Carstensen, (n. 15), I:501. See the chapter by George Zografi in this volume for information on the later development of the administration of the School.
25. Frederick B. Power, "The School of Pharmacy," in *The Badger Pharmacist* (Madison, 1900), 113.
26. *Ibid.*, 115–116.

27. *Ibid.*, 114; *First Annual Announcement of the Department of Pharmacy of the University of Wisconsin*, 1883–84, 2. There are copies of the early announcements of the Department of Pharmacy in the KRF under C31(a):I:Wisconsin.

28. Curti and Carstensen, (n. 15), I:352–354; *Dictionary of Wisconsin Biography* (Madison, 1960), 94; Aaron J. Ihde, *Chemistry, as Viewed from Bascom's Hill: A History of the Chemistry Department of the University of Wisconsin in Madison* (Madison, 1990), 58–63.

29. Kirtley Mather, "Charles Richard Van Hise," in *Dictionary of Scientific Biography* (New York, 1970–80; 16 vols.), XIII:572–573; Curti and Carstensen, (n. 15), II:3–122; Allen Debus, ed., *World Who's Who in Science* (Chicago, 1968), 1710; *Catalogue. . . Wisconsin*, 1883–84, p. 8; *Annual Announcement of the Department of Pharmacy of the University of Wisconsin*, various editions; Ihde, *Chemistry*, (n.28), 85–86, 102–103, 209–233.

30. Curti and Carstensen, (n. 15), I:361–362; Joseph Ewan, "William Trelease," in *Dictionary*, (n. 29), XIII:456.

31. Curti and Carstensen, (n. 15), I:355; *Dictionary*, (n.28), 97; Ihde, (n. 28), 54–58.

32. *Annual Announcement. . .* , various editions; *Catalogue*, 1883–84, 42; *ibid.*, 1884–85, 42. The manuscript notebooks of pharmacy student Henry Ruenzel for 1883–84 for the courses in botany, chemistry and pharmacy record the names of Power, Trelease, Daniells and Van Hise as instructors, but make no mention of Davies. These notebooks are in the KRF under C31(a)1:Wisconsin.

33. Power, "School," in *The Badger Pharmacist*, (n. 25), 113, "Report of Committee on School of Pharmacy," *Proc. WPhA.*, 4(1883):40–41; *ibid.*, 5(1884):40–42; *Annual Announcement*, 1883–84, 87.

34. Power, "School," in *The Badger Pharmacist*, (n. 25), 113.

35. *Annual Announcement*, 1883–84, 3; *ibid.*, 1884–85, 5; *Catalogue*, 1883–84, 87; *Annual Announcement of the School of Pharmacy of the University of Michigan*, 1883–84, 5; *Annual Announcement of the Philadelphia College of Pharmacy*, 1883, inside front cover.

36. *Annual Announcement*, 1883–83, 4; *ibid.*, 1884–85, 6; Sonnedecker, *History*, (n. 1), 236.

37. *Annual Announcement*, 1884–85, pp. 7–12; [Kremers], "Power," (n.16), 5–6; *Catalogue. . . Wisconsin*, 1883–84, 42; *ibid.*, 1884–85, 42.

38. *Annual Announcement. . . Michigan*, 1883–84; *Annual Announcement. . . Philadelphia*, 1883.

39. Power, "School," (n. 25), 118.

40. *Annual Announcement*, 1883–84, 5–6; *Annual Announcement. . . Michigan*, 1883–84, 12; *Annual Announcement. . . Philadelphia*, 1883, 22. On the ties between the Wisconsin Pharmaceutical Association and the University's pharmacy program during its early years, see Bardell, (n. 11), 15–23.

41. "Report of Committee," *Proc. WPhA.*, 5 (1884):40; "Wisconsin College of Pharmacy," *Drugg. Circ.*, 27(1883):122.

42. *Wisconsin State Journal*, Oct. 1 1883, 4; *ibid.*, Oct. 2, 1883, 4; "Report of Committee," *Proc. WPhA.*, 5 (1884): 40; notebooks of Henry Ruenzel, in KRF. Although the School of Pharmacy officially opened on October 1, it would appear that the first lectures were held the next day. Presumably the first day was devoted to registration and orientation of the students.

43. *Catalogue*, 1883–84, 21–22; *Annual Announcement*, 1884–85, 16; F. B. Power, "Report of the Professor of Pharmacy and Materia Medica," in *Biennial Report of the Board of Regents of the University of Wisconsin*, 1884, 47; untitled, undated two-page typescript listing students in first pharmacy class at Wisconsin "according to Professor Power's 'Record,'" in KRF under C31(a)I:Wisconsin. There is some discrepancy in the literature concerning the exact number of students enrolled in the first pharmacy class, but the best evidence seems to support the figure of 28. It is not clear, however, whether three or four of these students were enrolled as seniors. There were apparently also a few non-pharmacy students at the University who attended one or another of the pharmacy lecture courses and Power designated them as "elective" students. See the one-page typescript labelled "Electives," undated, in the KRF under C31(a):I:Wisconsin.

CHAPTER 2

Administration & Resources

BY GEORGE ZOGRAFI

WHAT FACTORS make a great educational institution? Excellent faculty? Outstanding students? Forward-thinking administrators? Material resources? The answer, of course, is all of the above, for a school can only be as good as the people who operate within its walls and the resources made available to carry out its programs. In this chapter we focus on some of the administrative factors that played a major role in the development of the School of Pharmacy. This includes the leadership it received, its place within the University structure, the financial and other resources made available, and the interrelationships which developed between the School and various pharmacy groups within the State of Wisconsin.

For present purposes it is convenient to divide the School's first century into five periods. In the *first period* we have the administration of F. B. Power from 1883 to 1892, the time from the founding of the School, to a point where its place in the University was reasonably well established. It was a period which, despite limited resources, brought slow and steady improvement in student enrollment, while beginning to create a climate of quality instruction and scholarship.

In the *second period* from 1892 to about 1918, under the leadership of Edward Kremers, dramatic and unprecedented changes took place in the degree programs offered, the general standards of instruction and the level of scholarship and research. To say that this period was revolutionary and long-lasting in its effects would not be an overstatement.

From 1918 to about 1950, under the leadership of Kremers (until 1935), and Arthur H. Uhl after that, came the *third period*. This was a time that brought significant growth in enrollments, after the low enrollments of the previous period, and a slow but steady strengthening of undergraduate and graduate programs. It was a period when resources, needed to take

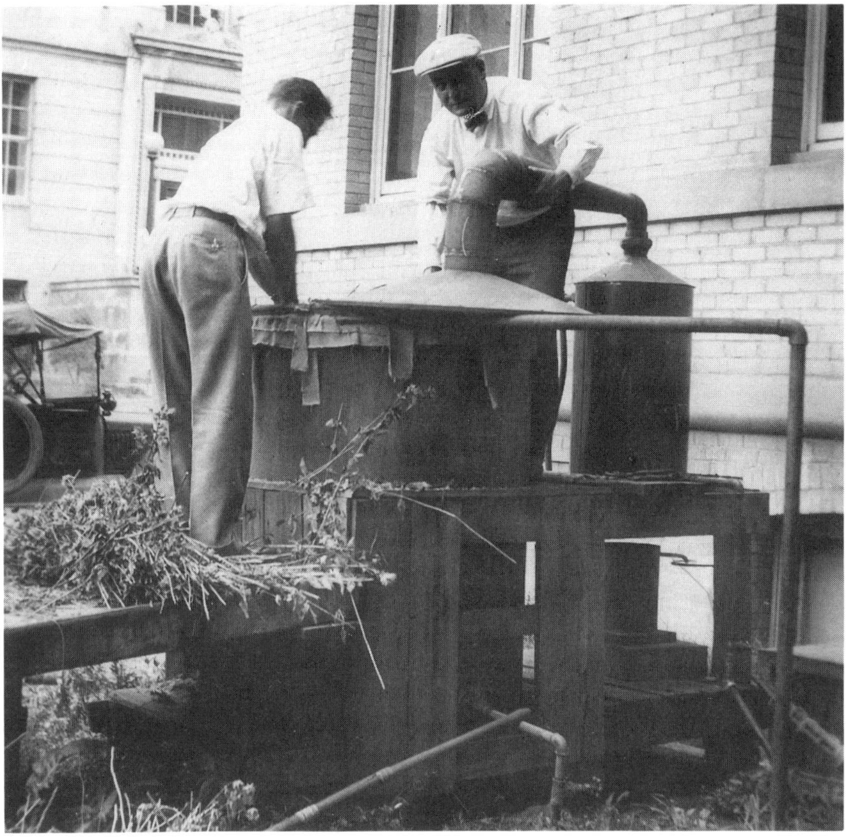

Harvest time in the acreage of medicinal plants kept the steam still busy outside the School of Pharmacy during the flourishing years of the Pharmaceutical Experiment Station (1913–35).

advantage of the earlier changes, were not as available as had been hoped for, due in part to the economic depression in the 1930s, followed by the period of World War II.

The *fourth period* covered the years 1950–68, under the leadership of Uhl, who became the first dean of the newly independent School of Pharmacy. This period coincided with the unprecedented economic growth in this country after War II, along with a significant demand for pharmacy graduates at the B.Sc. and post-B.Sc. levels. During this time a more modern curriculum was developed; graduate programs grew in size and impact; Extension Services in Pharmacy became a major educational program; and an innovative pharmacy internship program within the State of Wisconsin was developed. In all respects it was a period of great significance in reaffirming a central role for Wisconsin in pharmaceutical education and the pharmaceutical sciences.

The *fifth period*, from 1968 into the start of a second century, brought the School under the leadership of five deans: David Perlman (1968–75); George Zografi (1975–80); August P. Lemberger (1980–90); Donald T. Witiak (1993–95); Melvin H. Weinswig (1995–); and an interim dean, Kenneth A. Connors (1990–93). For biographic portraits of the deans that served during the School's first century, see *Appendix 1* (p. 169).

The rapid change that marked this fifth period was brought about primarily by factors external to the University. It started with significant increases in faculty size and greater state resources to accommodate large increases in undergraduate enrollments and the development of additional degree programs (see chapters 3 and 5). This was accompanied by increased support of the federal government in the form of biomedical research grants to the faculty and the "capitation" grants for the improvement of undergraduate programs, including the development of a new clinical pharmacy program. This led to a much larger total faculty and staff than ever before. Towards the end of this period, however, there was a change in the national economic situation, which led to the federal and state governments pulling back in the level of their support for the University.

Administrative Structure Within the University

When Power first opened the doors of the Department of Pharmacy, the University's structure was relatively uncomplicated, because of its small size. Pharmacy itself had 28 students among a total University enrollment of 388, 7% of the total (contrasting with about 1% a century later). Because of the relatively small scale on which everything operated, Power had ready access to the President of the University and the Board of Regents when important administrative matters arose.

During the last decades of the nineteenth century a number of special schools were created within the University. These included economics and political science, history, commerce, and education. As the University grew in numbers of faculty and students, and as the different types of disciplines presenting instruction increased in number, the administration of the University became more complex, and a need to be more organized seemed apparent to the University administration. President Van Hise therefore undertook a change in administrative structure in 1903, apparently without much prior consultation,[1] in essence, placing the various "schools" mentioned above, including the Department of Pharmacy, under the administrative supervision of the Dean of the College of Letters and Sciences (labeled as "Courses in . . . "). For Pharmacy this arrangement was to last until 1950; although as early as 1916, the Wisconsin Pharmaceutical Association's School of Pharmacy Committee called for the establishment of an independent college of pharmacy with its own dean.[2]

Although much progress in education and research was made by the School during these years, it is clear that Edward Kremers, who directed the School during most of this period, was disturbed by the situation.[3] Of critical importance to him, and to his successor in 1935, Arthur H. Uhl, was their inability to develop a direct relationship with the President of the University, rather than having to bring all administrative matters first to the Dean of Letters and Sciences. Of concern also was the minimal flexibility permitted in dealing with problems as they arose, and the fact that decisions were being made without a good understanding of the needs unique to Pharmacy. In 1939 the Department of Pharmacy was officially designated a School within the College of Letters and Science; but the lack of full status as a professional school, along the lines of medicine and law, was seen by Kremers as an impediment to the promotion of the profession. After World War II, Wisconsin was perhaps the only School of Pharmacy in an American university lacking independent status. The American Council on Pharmaceutical Education, in its accreditation report of 1949[4], stated, "The committee also is inclined to raise the question as to whether or not the subordinate position in which the School of

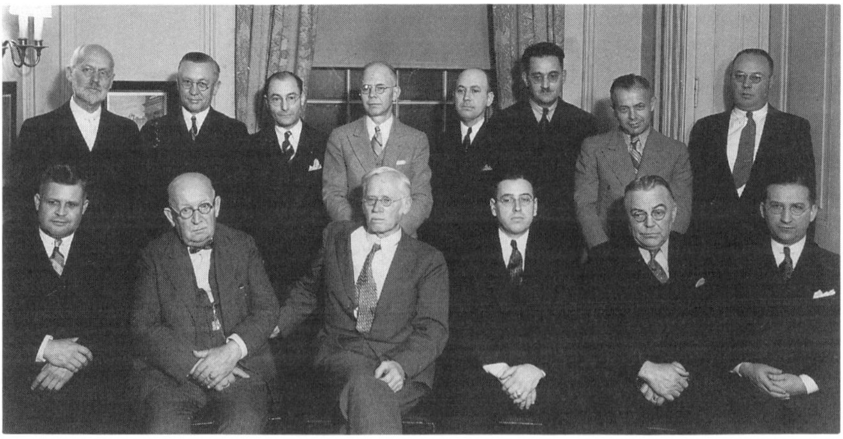

Meetings between representatives of the pharmacy faculty, the Wisconsin Pharmaceutical Association, and the State Board of Pharmacy, as shown in this 1938 conference, fostered cooperation. The participants were: (top, l. to r.) W.O. Richtmann, Oscar Rennebohm, Wilbur C. Lalis, Bruno F. Leidel, Jennings Murphy, Edwin J. Boberg, William Rhyme, and Ralph Clark; (bottom, l. to r.) John Huber, Henry Ruenzel, Edward Kremers, Arthur H. Uhl, B.J. Kremer, and S.H. Dretzka.

Pharmacy is placed in the university organization may be a contributing factor in unduly retarding its progress."

While this administrative structure existed, periodic calls for independent status were made by committee reports and resolutions from the Wisconsin Pharmaceutical Association, but were given no serious consideration until 1948–49, when the faculty and WPhA met on several occasions to develop approaches to the problem. This culminated in a letter from the WPhA to the University's President, E. B. Fred, on March 14, 1949, requesting consideration of independent status and citing numerous reasons for this request.[5] WPhA also worked to introduce a bill into the Wisconsin State Legislature which permitted the University to establish an independent School of Pharmacy.

President Fred responded quickly to the calls for action, establishing a University committee to consider the matter (March 28, 1949). Included as members were: Vice President for Academic Affairs, I. L. Baldwin; Dean of the College of Letters and Sciences, M. H. Ingraham; Dean of the Medical School, W. S. Middleton; Professor of Chemistry, S. M. McElvain; and Director of the School of Pharmacy, A. H. Uhl. In June of 1949, the Committee presented its report[6], recommending establishment of an independent school, with two members, Ingraham and McElvain, both from the College of Letters and Sciences, recommending postponement until a two-year prepharmacy requirement within their College could be developed. In 1950 the Board of Regents established the School, with a one-year prepharmacy course sequence within the four-year baccalaureate program. From remarks made later by President Fred it is clear that a major concern of the College of Letters of Sciences was an erosion of its influence in higher administrative matters by the presence of many smaller independent schools.[7]

From 1950 into the 1970s the School of Pharmacy experienced unprecedented growth in faculty, students, and resources, as well as significant national and international renown as a major center of pharmaceutical research and education. It was a period when the emphasis on basic scientific principles, instilled by Power and Kremers in the early years, was being rediscovered by national pharmaceutical educators, and when, because of its tradition, the School was again able to assume a strong leadership role, particularly in the basic areas of pharmaceutical chemistry, biochemistry, pharmacology, physical pharmacy, pharmacy administration, and the history of pharmacy.

At the same time the nature of health care in this country, and particularly the role to be played by various health professionals, began to

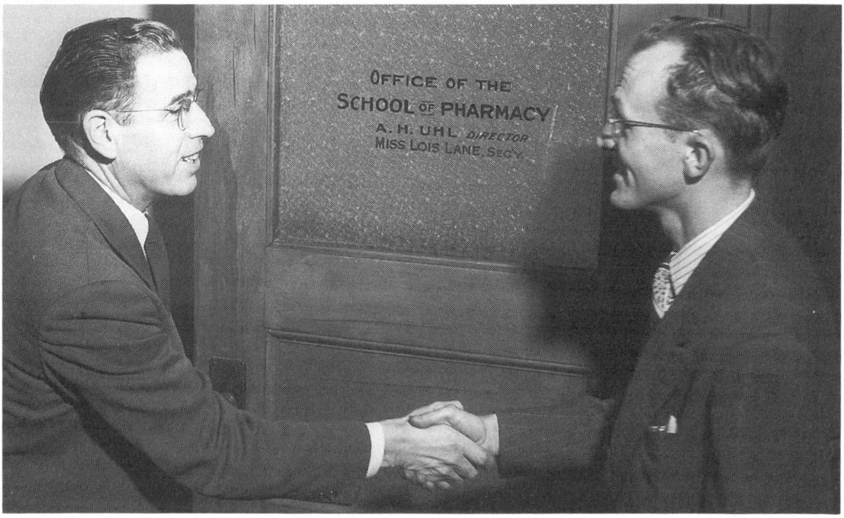
OFFICE OF THE
SCHOOL OF PHARMACY
A. H. UHL DIRECTOR
MISS LOIS LANE, SEC'Y.

Dean Arthur Uhl welcomes to his office in the late 1940s a graduate student, Gordon Svoboda, who later became a prominent researcher in the Lilly laboratories. As an administrator, Uhl was exceptionally sympathetic to students' hopes and concerns.

surface as an important national issue. With the practicing pharmacist no longer a major factor in the compounding and manufacture of pharmaceutical products, organized pharmacy was reexamining its role in the health-care system. A strong national consensus emerged that the future of pharmacy as an essential service to the patient rested on its ability to impact on the clinical use of drugs in addition to its more traditional role.[8] This concept of "clinical pharmacy" coincided with a more general interest on the part of universities in bringing their various health-profession schools closer together, so as to encourage greater joint effort in the delivery of health care, research, and teaching. Thus, many universities in the 1960s established new administrative units known as centers of health science, combining schools of medicine, pharmacy, nursing, dentistry, and other health professions.

In 1970, after establishing a School of Allied Health Professions, the University of Wisconsin in Madison organized a new administrative unit, the Center for Health Sciences, under the leadership of a Vice Chancellor who reported directly to the Chancellor of the University. This unit was set up to consist of the Medical School; the Schools of Pharmacy, of Nursing, and of Allied Health Professions; the Student Health Service; The University Hospital and Clinics; The State Laboratory of Hygiene; and the Wisconsin Psychiatric Institute. Initially there was great reluctance on the part of the School of Pharmacy faculty and administration (as well as some of the other schools) to become part of another administrative unit, and particularly to become budgetarily linked to other schools with competing interests.[9] It appeared too similar to the pre–1950 period when the School was administered by the College of Letters and Sciences. There also were many who saw this development as leading to a break with related basic sciences, particularly if the entire Center for Health Sciences was eventually to be housed together in a separate part of the campus.[10] On the positive side, the structure was seen as offering the School of Pharmacy an opportunity to become more intimately involved in health care in its teaching and research programs. Moreover, it should be able to bring its basic science expertise to bear more directly on important health-related problems, through collaborative multidisciplinary teaching and research.

The Center for Health Sciences evolved to a point where the general role it would play became clearer. Direct access by deans to the Chancellor remained available. However, the Vice Chancellor, who met regularly with the Chancellor and other top administrators, provided a convenient channel of communication from and to the School. Budgetary activity proceeded directly from the School to the Chancellor's office, with the Vice Chancellor playing an advisory role in the process. The Vice Chancellor and the Center also facilitated communications and activity among various health units within the Center. This included joint efforts in the development of such Center-wide programs as geriatric health care, emergency medical care, clinical nutrition, and toxicology, as well as the formation of Center-wide committees such as curriculum, radiation safety, and human experimentation. The Center, through the Vice Chancellor, played an important role in representing all of the health schools to state government and to other state and national agencies related to health care. But during the 1990s an increased role would again emerge for Deans of the component schools in coordinating activities.

Faculty Structure and Governance

Within this general picture of how the School of Pharmacy was administratively situated within the larger University, how did it function internally during various periods in its history and what kind of leadership did it receive? As can be seen from the listing of faculty members who have served the School (see *Appendix* 2), the size of School faculty relative to the rest of the University faculty, or even relative to many of the major departments on campus, has always been quite small. During the nine years that F. B. Power was professor and director, the School had no faculty of its own except for Power and Edward Kremers, who joined the staff as a laboratory instructor in 1889. From the beginning, Power was intent on developing something different for pharmacy at this School, along the lines Professor Flückiger had developed at the University of Strassburg.[11] He saw state support for education versus the independent schools' reliance on student fees as an opportunity for Wisconsin to strengthen pharmaceutical education.[12]

In assessing this period it is clear that Power was content to move slowly in building his program and developing relations with the pharmacists of the state, before making dramatic moves, though he had a strong interest in scholarship. For example, in contrast to the University of Michigan, where apprenticeship experience was not required for admission, Power opted to retain the common practice of two years apprenticeship before the abbreviated two-year sequence of courses for the Ph.G. degree. He expressed a desire that students have a high school diploma as a requirement for admission to the program, but it was not until much

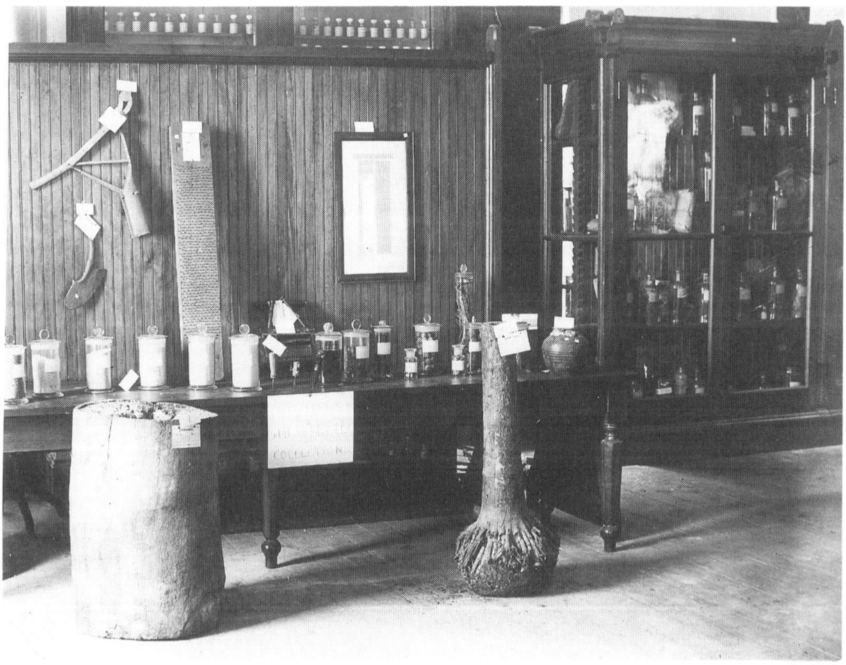

A materia medica collection of about five thousand specimens from around the world, pride of the School by the turn of the century, was relegated to the attic sometime after the 1930s and later contributed to the Smithsonian Institution.

later under Kremers that this actually was to happen. Thus he was capable of compromise on occasion in order to build a program having the characteristics and quality he sought. However, in later writings by Kremers,[13] there is a strong indication that Power was not pleased with the level of support he received from the University and the pharmacists and that this was the main reason that he left "in disgust" to assume another position. Yet, we find no indication of this in Power's own writings. It seems clear that his leadership put the School in a forward position in pharmaceutical education at that time, particularly because of his insistence on laboratory instruction and research, and his high standards and expectation of the students. As early as 1890, for example an extensive review of the University of Wisconsin School of Pharmacy in the *Pharmaceutische Rundschau*[14] emphasized how much the School had been able to accomplish in only seven years.

In 1892, when Power left the University and Edward Kremers, then only 27 years old, assumed his position, many changes took place almost immediately. (On Kremers, see also p. 171.) Specific accomplishments of Kremers and the School of Pharmacy in education and research in the next few decades will be addressed in other chapters, but here we should at least get some feeling for the general situation during this period.

By 1900 Kremers had upgraded the pharmacy faculty considerably. Although he remained the only full-time PhD on the faculty, his roster listed a dozen PhD's drawn from other UW departments who were teaching pharmacy students part-time, plus an instructor (PhC, MD) and student assistants. This was remarkable at that period in American pharmaceutical education. By 1895 he was able to establish five "distinctively" pharmaceutical departments of instruction: pharmaceutical chemistry, pharmaceutical botany, pharmaceutical techniques, pharmacognosy and practical pharmacy. Although these were called departments there is no indication of such status officially, nor did Kremers ever delegate budgetary authority to these groups. Much later, in 1925, the faculty size at the instructorship and professorial level was reduced by one, compared to 1900, with much more use being made of graduate-student assistance. At that time only Dr. W. O. Richtmann and Dr. Nellie Wakeman were at the Assistant Professor level. Although there was no formal administrative structure in the School below the level of Director, Richtmann was delegated as early as 1926 to act on behalf of Kremers in his absence.[15]

There is no evidence of formal and regular faculty meetings where minutes were taken. Kremers ran his department in the classic European style, where the "Professor" was the dominant figure in all respects. He determined educational policy, supervised all scholarly activity, aggressively represented the school to the University administration and to the Wisconsin Pharmaceutical Association, and was a prominent figure at the national and international level. In contrast to Power, he was very forceful and often impatient with situations that unnecessarily delayed reform, not holding back in his criticism of WPhA members when he felt the School was being treated unfairly. He had a religious fervor concerning pharmacy and the standards it must attain to join its "sister professions" in stature. For example, he once referred to the Wisconsin state motto "Forward," when speaking with pride of the School's accomplishments.[16] We cannot know whether he would have been even more effective as an administrator, in gaining financial support and physical facilities, had he possessed greater diplomacy. Those working on the faculty might have gained enhanced reputations of their own if Kremers had not been so dominant; but there is no doubt of the quality of those who were trained by him, and there can be no doubt of the lasting impact he had on the School of Pharmacy and the profession of pharmacy as well.

In 1935, Kremers retired and Assistant Professor Arthur H. Uhl (see p. 173) assumed leadership of the School, which by now had an in-house

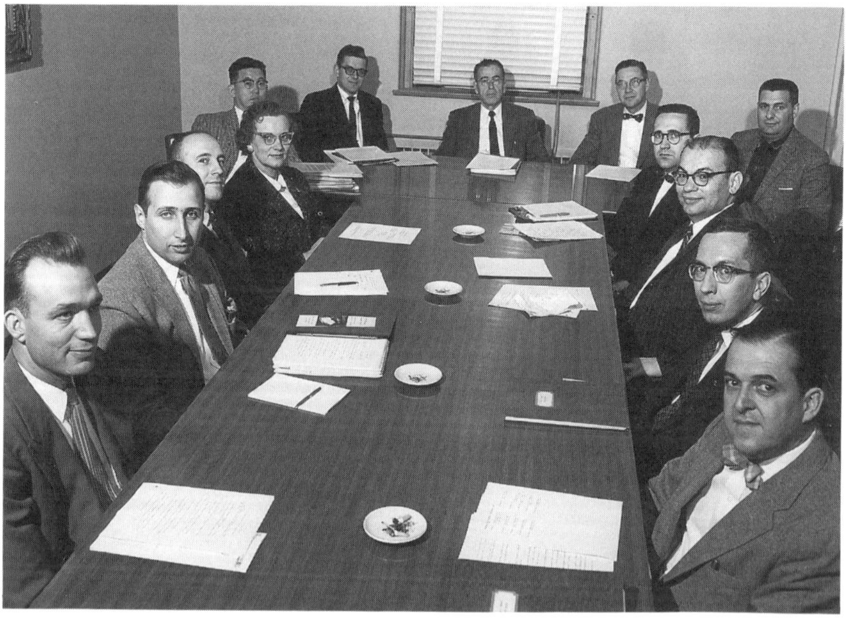

School policies have been influenced by faculty deliberations over the decades. A rare view of a faculty meeting is this photo from the late 1950s, showing (l. to r.): Jack Miller, Hyman Mitchner, W. Allen Daniels, Eunice Bonow, Takeru Higuchi, August P. Lemberger, Arthur H. Uhl (Dean and chair), Louis W. Busse, William S. Apple (away from table), Edward Smissman, Morris Kupchan, Joseph Cannon, and Dale Wurster.

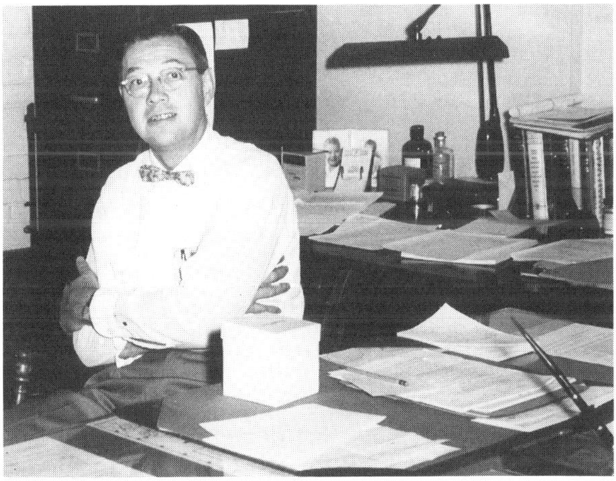

Professor Louis W. Busse in 1954, when he became the first Associate Dean. Busse had a major role in the administration of the School and, nationally, in affairs of the AACP.

faculty consisting only of Uhl, Wakeman, Richtmann and an instructor, Ralph Clark. The transition apparently was somewhat complicated by the continuing presence of Uhl's predecessor (until his death in 1941), given Kremers' personality and style. From the beginning, however, the tone of the administration changed significantly. For example, as early as 1939, Uhl was holding regular monthly faculty meetings and beginning to develop better communications with the pharmacists of the state. In other respects, until the end of World War II, the School operated much as in previous years, but in most dimensions on a much smaller scale.

The post-war period under Uhl was a dynamic period of growth and accomplishment. From 1939 to 1948, the faculty grew from five full-time individuals to seven, but by 1952, shortly after the School attained independent status, there were 10 individuals of professorial rank, and before Uhl retired in 1968, the faculty had grown to a professorial group of about 24.

Minutes of the faculty meetings, which generally were held on Saturday morning, tell us that under Uhl there was a significant amount of faculty involvement in the operation of the program. In 1948, for example, eight faculty committees were functioning: curriculum, library, student organizations, alumni relations, placement (for employment of students), publicity, and Pharmacy ROTC, as well as an executive committee of four members selected by Uhl. In 1954 the School added an Associate Dean, Dr. Louis W. Busse. By 1963 there was only one more committee, but six of the nine had titles and tasks different from the 1948 list, namely: admissions, building, citations, scholarships and awards, library, lectures, graduate study, curriculum and a six-person executive committee.

In reviewing the faculty minutes during the immediate post-war period one is struck particularly by the characteristics of the individuals who served on the faculty during this time. Strong willed and bright individuals like Lloyd Parks, Louis Busse, George Urdang, Takeru Higuchi, Dale Wurster, William Apple, Joseph Swintosky, and Glenn Sonnedecker must have played a significant role in addressing the needs of the School and the profession during that period. Uhl is known to have remarked, on many occasions, that he saw his role as one of "finding outstanding faculty and then staying out of their way."[17] From the recollections of some,[18] it appears that Uhl was particularly effective in his relationships with pharmacists, alumni, and students and that he spent considerable time developing and nurturing such relationships. He left much of the administration of the School to his Associate Dean, Louis Busse, and the rest of the faculty and was not aggressively involved in University-wide affairs. Thus this period must be considered one where faculty initiatives predominated, guided by the receptive leadership of Uhl (in contrast to the Kremers era) in bringing about significant accomplishments.

As the School entered the latter half of the 1960s, at its peak of educational and research activity, the social structure of society was starting to change rapidly. This was brought on in part by a greater awareness of social problems in this country and a greater tendency, particularly of young people, to speak out and demonstrate against the established norms of that period. The Vietnam War surfaced as a focal point of this "protest period" in the late 1960s, but even earlier changes in the tastes of youth in music and dress and hair styles were symptomatic of a dramatic change in society. The University of Wisconsin in Madison certainly felt the impact of this changing social situation, as it had felt other such changes during its history. The "post-Sputnik" period brought a rapid expansion in research support from federal sources, increased support for Ph.D. graduates in the sciences, badly in short supply, and increased state funds to support many of the programs needed to meet these demands. It was a period of "big science" and a demand for aggressive research activity, to which the School of Pharmacy was in relatively good position to respond in pharmacy, pharmaceutical chemistry and pharmacognosy, but less so in pharmacology and biomedically-related research.

This is the situation that Dr. David Perlman (see p. 175) encountered as he became the fourth head of the School of Pharmacy in 1968, after Uhl reached retirement age. Indeed, Perlman's first two years in office had to contend with reflections of the times such as a University-wide strike of teaching assistants, a Pharmacy School dress-code dispute, and a Vietnam-War protest bombing next door to the School, which did about $1,000,000 worth of damage to the School's facilities. Within the School of Pharmacy at this time a significant increase in undergraduate enrollments created a corresponding need for staff, space and equipment, to which Perlman addressed much of his attention.

The need for more administrative assistance was apparent, and it was during this period that two Assistant Deans, one for professional and student affairs, Dr. Richard Ohvall, and the other for graduate studies and research, Dr. Kenneth Connors, were appointed. In 1970, when Ohvall left to assume a deanship elsewhere, his position was elevated to that of Associate Dean and was filled by Dr. Melvin Weinswig, who also served as Chairman of Extension Services in Pharmacy. From 1972 to 1974, Dr. Philip Hart assumed the position of Assistant Dean for graduate studies. During the tenure of Dean Perlman (1968 to 1975) he was able to expand the faculty and staff, preside over an expansion of the physical plant, increase research support from extramural sources, and significantly increase the School's budget.

Faculty participation in governance, which had become generally more formalized in the University during the 1960s, also became more formalized at the School in the Perlman years. In 1968, for example, Perlman expanded the membership and role of the Executive Committee. All tenured faculty were included, as was the practice in other departments of the University, and were charged with the responsibility of all academic personnel review as well as budget review. This fresh approach to faculty governance in the School continued into the 1980s with success. During this period, through the expansion of the pharmacology program, the greater involvement of the School in the Center for Health Sciences, and the increased interactions with the University Hospital because of the introduction of clinical teaching to pharmacy students, the visibility of the School and its faculty as both a resource in biomedical research and representing pharmacy as a health-care profession, increased significantly, although Dean Perlman always was uncomfortable with the possibility of pharmacy subordinating its identity to the Medical School, its larger partner in the Center for Health Sciences.[19]

After Perlman resigned to return to full-time teaching and research in 1975, his successors during the rest of the first century, Deans George Zografi (1975–80) and August Lemberger (1980–90)—see pages 177–180—

continued the over-all pattern of administration within the School. Zografi appointed four part-time Assistant Deans, from the faculty: W. M. Dickson, G. L. Amidon, D. H. Rich, and P. G. Welling. Lemberger changed this structure, in 1980–81, by appointing an Associate Dean for graduate studies, Bonnie Svarstad; and later, William Mellon—and as Associate Dean for student and professional affairs, C. A. Bond. Two challenging situations emerged during the final period here discussed, especially after the early

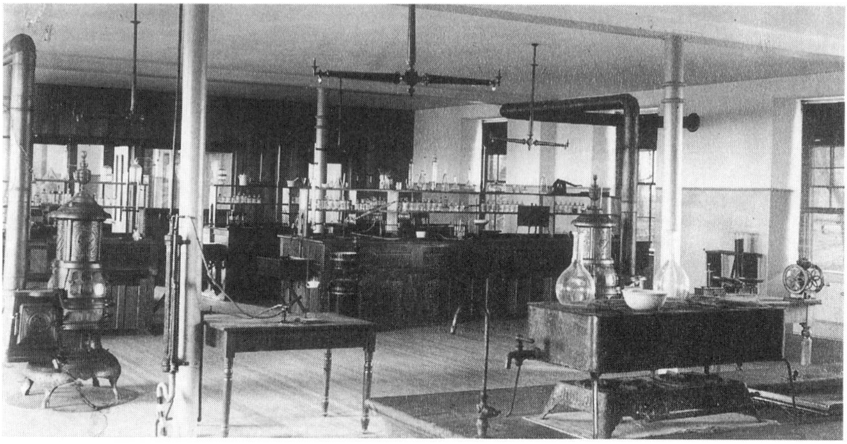

The pharmaceutical laboratory of the School in 1890 provided experience in small-scale manufacture, emphasizing galenicals.

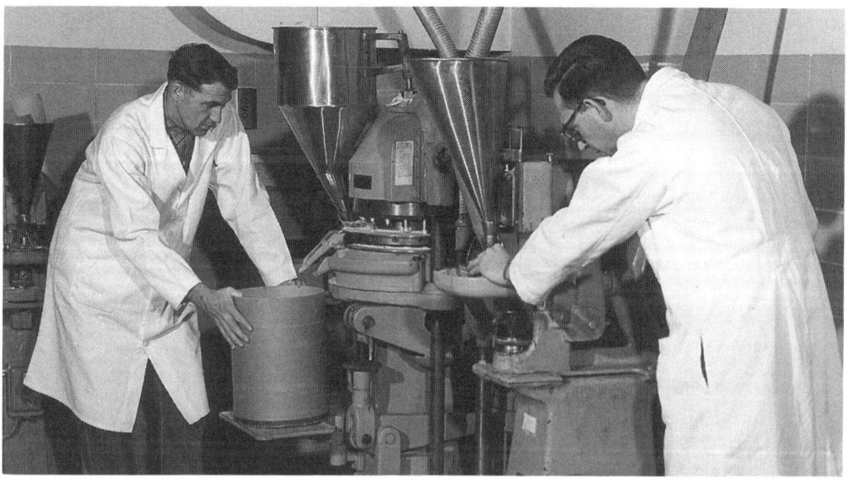

Drug manufacturing facilities, partly shown in this 1957 photograph, had been enhanced through the School's commitment to supply various medications to University Hospitals and other state institutions for their patients.

1970s: First the deteriorating economic situation in Wisconsin and nationally, and the slow elimination of federal funding to Schools of Pharmacy, severely constrained the School from expanding various activities to meet perceived program needs. Second, the need to develop clinical instruction in pharmacy became not only apparent, but became a requirement for continued accreditation.[20] By 1975 it was apparent that greater attention to the development of clinical instruction, faculty and sites was required. Utilizing capitation funds and reallocating resources in the absence of new state funds, attempts were made to enlarge the full-time clinical faculty, to make better use of the pharmacy staffs of the University Hospital and Veterans Administration to develop a clerkship with extended block periods for greater student contact in both outpatient and inpatient settings, and to set up criteria for allowing clinical research to be carried out by various clinical faculty. By 1982, much progress had been made in attaining these goals, as the clinical staff numbered 11 clinical professors and 16 clinical instructors.

Physical Facilities

One recurring theme during the first century of this School's existence, besides independent status, was the desire for more space and for a separate School of Pharmacy building.

The description of Power's first sight of his facilities in South Hall (page 22) provides a vivid glimpse of the humble beginnings experienced by pharmacy on the Madison campus. In 1889, as the pharmacy program developed and enrollments grew, it was necessary for the School to move to North Hall, where it occupied the third and fourth floors. Despite the increased space there, some indication of discontent with these facilities was expressed by the pharmacists of the state as early as 1900 when they resolved at the WPhA meeting, "that this Association request that a sufficient sum be donated to build a building on University grounds for the Department of Pharmacy and that the committee of legislation push the matter during the session of the Legislature."[21]

Edward Kremers acknowledged the inadequate facilities in North Hall and the desirability of a new separate building. However, in his quest for improving the quality and standards of the program he often appeared to play down the inadequacy of the facilities. For example, during one such discussion related to the issue of facilities he quoted the late Professor van Hoffman by saying "the cage is immaterial, the question is whether the bird in the cage can sing."[22]

Following a period of rapid growth of the University, the state legislature in 1903 appropriated $100,000 for a new chemical building at the corner of University Avenue and North Charter Street, and it was in this building that the School of Pharmacy would remain into its second century. In 1913, an addition to the chemical building was constructed, but there is no evidence that the School gained new space. The move to the chemical building may have played some role in strengthening the natural ties that exist between chemistry and pharmacy; but throughout the years, evidence suggests that the School of Pharmacy, the smaller unit, had great difficulty getting the space it thought it required. In 1924, for example, the WPhA Committee on the School of Pharmacy reported that "there was a crying need for space in the chemical building." They further strongly suggested that the time had come again to press for a separate building.[23] Indeed, a legislative bill was put forth in 1926 to fund a separate building, but it failed to pass (in one person's opinion because there was little support expressed by the pharmacists of the state at the public hearing).[24] In 1927 $350,000 were allocated for a new wing of the chemical building, and Pharmacy did receive some limited additional space to house the F. B. Power Library, the Drug Cabinet (a valuable collection of specimens previously in storage), one small research laboratory, and a new dispensing laboratory. In 1930, however, strong disappointment with this situation was expressed at the annual WPhA meeting.[25] It was felt that if the $350,000 had been given to Pharmacy, Chemistry would have had the vacated space within its building, which it required, and Pharmacy would have its own badly needed separate facility.

Little further mention was made of the need for physical facilities as the economic depression arrived, followed by World War II. It was not until 1945, when the University in general began to update its physical plant to meet the demands of post-war growth, that mention of a new building once again appears. In its annual report of 1945, the WPhA Committee on the School of Pharmacy recognized the need to link fund-raising for a new pharmacy building with the general University building campaign.[26] It even recommended the use of Association funds to draw up preliminary architectural sketches of a possible building.

In 1947, after considerable activity by the School administration and WPhA, Lawrence F. Madland, a Milwaukee alumnus who chaired the School of Pharmacy Building Committee, could report that $192,000 had been allocated to renovate the Chemistry Building, including parts of the third and fourth floor occupied by Pharmacy, and that an entire new wing on the northwest side of the building would be constructed when funds became available.[27] Indeed, in 1955, the School of Pharmacy was able to expand into a new $380,000 addition to the Chemistry Building, with its own entrance identified at 425 Charter Street. The new construction contained four floors of laboratories and offices, plus a basement and subbasement, the latter being used as a manufacturing laboratory.

In addition to research laboratories for 56 graduate students working for doctoral degrees, the facility included an analytical laboratory operated with the State Board of Pharmacy for testing samples of various drug products taken from the field during inspections. Although this was not the independent facility long sought, it represented the first new permanent facility built expressly for the School of Pharmacy.

In the years that followed, the School of Pharmacy underwent significant growth in faculty and students, as did the Chemistry Department, with which it continued to share some space on the third and fourth floors of the old wings. Thus, the pressure for more space persisted. Already in 1958, for example, Pharmacy and Chemistry were discussing plans to renovate space in the older wing of the building, which would be made available by the planned construction of a new chemistry research building on West Johnson Street. The basic plan was to seek funds from the National

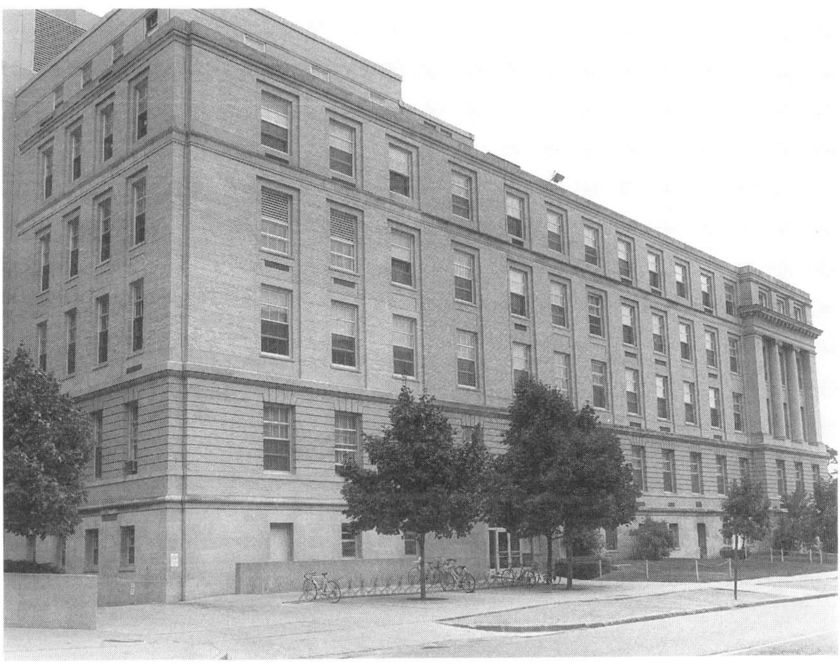

Pharmacy expanded its facilities when an addition (at left) to the west wing of the building opened in 1955. The main entrance shifted to Charter Street, giving the School a visual identity on-campus for the first time.

Institutes of Health, Wisconsin Alumni Research Foundation and the State of Wisconsin for a "research wing" to be shared by Pharmacy; and part of the Chemistry Department would be left behind until a *second* phase of the new chemistry facility on Johnson Street could be built. There was some tension between the two units over the amount of space to be allocated, and this plan did not materialize.[28]

During the 1960s the need for physical facilities and plans to secure new quarters continued to be a major issue in the School faculty, leading to some improvement in the amount of space allocated, but also leading to disappointment with regard to the development of separate facilities. With the projected move of the Chemistry Department, a number of factors triggered much action. The University decided early that the oldest part of the building (the center section) would require complete renovation and that the Physics Department would be allotted much of the space vacated by Chemistry. At the time, Pharmacy had about 50,000 sq. ft. of space, some of it in the center section.

In the period 1965–67, therefore, discussions turned toward constructing a separate 90,000 sq. ft. building for Pharmacy, but the University administration countered with a proposal for a two-phase move, a new 40,000 sq. ft. building at University and Orchard Street to be built in Phase I and 50,000 sq. ft. to be added later as Phase II.[29] Reluctant acceptance of this approach by the pharmacy faculty led to elaborate plans for separating research and teaching facilities. In 1968, the new dean of the School, David Perlman, worked vigorously with the faculty and administration to obtain some resources from the federal government for such a building, then planned for a site at Brooks and Johnson Streets. After significant planning and effort, the grant was approved but *not* funded.

In 1970 at the peak of student opposition to the Vietnam War, extremists set off an explosion between the Army Mathematics Research Center in Sterling Hall and the School of Pharmacy, which caused damage of about $1-million to the School. Moreover, the central part of the building had to be razed, which led to some "temporary" moving around of pharmacy facilities. Most notably the School occupied space in the East Wing that originally had been allocated to Physics, but that department had undergone some enrollment declines and had less need for the space. During this time, the School of Pharmacy was undergoing significant growth in students, faculty, and research activity, and the pressures for space were enormous. When the dust had settled, the School found itself expanded to about 75,000 sq. ft. in the entire west wing and all but the top floor of the east wing, the latter going to the Medical School for an immunobiology

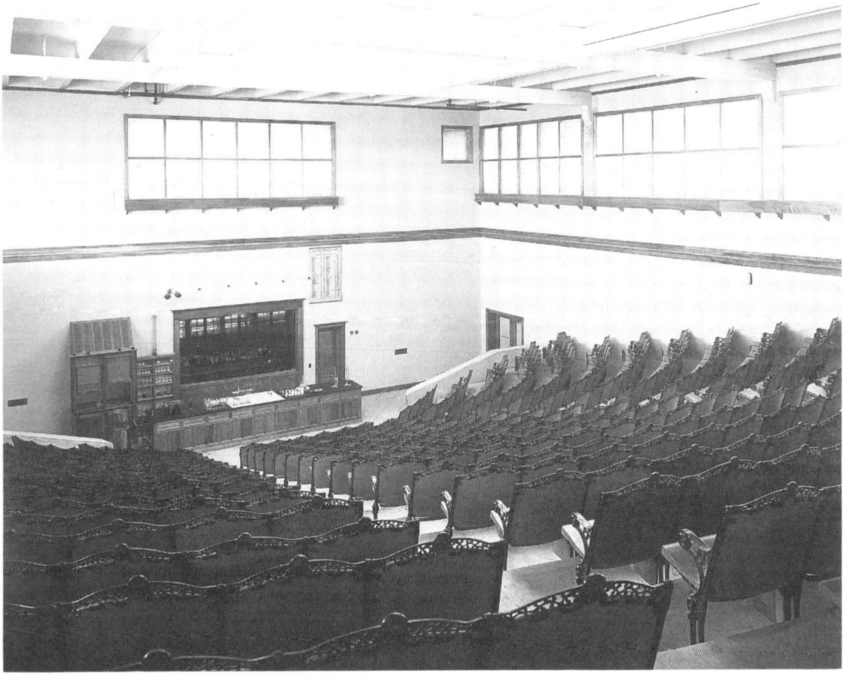

For generations of pharmacy students after the turn of the century, Chemistry 100 (above) was probably their most familiar classroom. It was replaced as the fulcrum of School activities when the Rennebohm Auditorium (below) was dedicated in 1978.

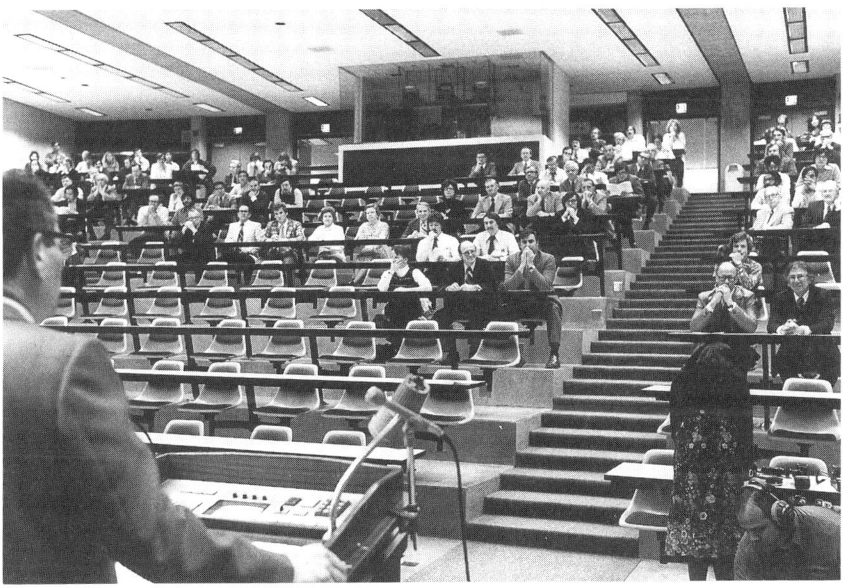

research center. The new center section was assigned to the Physics Department, continuing the division of the School into two parts.

After 1972 when the Chemistry Building, now called Chamberlin Hall, was renovated, it had become clear that the School would be housed in this facility for an indefinite period and not get its own building. Systematic efforts, therefore, were made each year to renovate various parts of the building, through federal, state and private funding. In 1978, for example, a new 250-seat auditorium was built in a subbasement of the east wing, with funds from all three sources. The private funds came from the Oscar Rennebohm Foundation and the auditorium was named after Mr. Rennebohm, who had been a successful pharmacist, former Governor of the State, Regent of the University and a very active worker in the WPhA toward attaining a new building and independent status for the School. But the old dream of a separate, adequate building was not to be fulfilled until well after the close of the first century.

Financial Resources

In addition to providing physical facilities for the use of faculty and students, a university must find the means to provide salaries for personnel, equipment for instruction and research and a library with a collection of some substance. Given the funds to provide such resources, a school or department has responsibility to use such funds wisely and effectively. By tradition at the University of Wisconsin, units such as the School of Pharmacy have been given significant flexibility in how funds are to be used, with the main basis of most state support being the instructional programs and the number of students enrolled in such programs.

A broad picture of resources generally made available to the School over the years is portrayed below to show how such resources have impacted on the ability of the School to develop its programs. Dollar amounts mentioned do not take into account inflation, hence are not directly comparable.

When the School was founded in 1883 a sum of $2,000 was provided to F. B. Power for salary and other expenses. The Wisconsin Pharmaceutical Association appears to have raised the funds necessary to print and distribute the announcement of the course prepared by Power.[30] Student laboratory fees were the primary source of funds for equipment and supplies. With the expansion of laboratory instruction and the addition of more staff in the 1890s the total state allocation increased to $7,500 by 1895–96, out of a total University budget of $404,600. Of that amount, $6,400 was used for salaries (including $2,000 for Edward Kremers' salary),

$270 for janitorial services, and $830 for equipment.[31] Approximately this level of instructional budget continued until about the early 1920s, probably due to limited change in enrollments (see *Appendix 4a*). In 1923–24, for example, the amount available for salaries from the instructional budget was only $10,900, in contrast to a budget for the Chemistry Department of $91,360 and for the Classics Department of $18,650. The budget of the Pharmaceutical Experimental Station[32] (see Chapter 5) eventually was used in part to pay some faculty salaries. As early as 1898, Kremers was expressing concern about the salaries he could offer faculty and the keen competition with other schools for qualified faculty.[33] This has been a chronic problem at the University of Wisconsin, which often has ranked relatively low in overall faculty salaries when compared to universities of similar scope and quality.

Budgets since World War II are not directly comparable because of inflation, but it is noteworthy that when the School first became independent in 1950, it had a budget of $102,725, of which $77,725 was for salaries, while in 1981–82 the total budget was $3,886,972, of which $2,558,554 was for salaries. These latter figures reflect much more than state-supported funds ($2,437,871), including funds from extramural sources, particularly

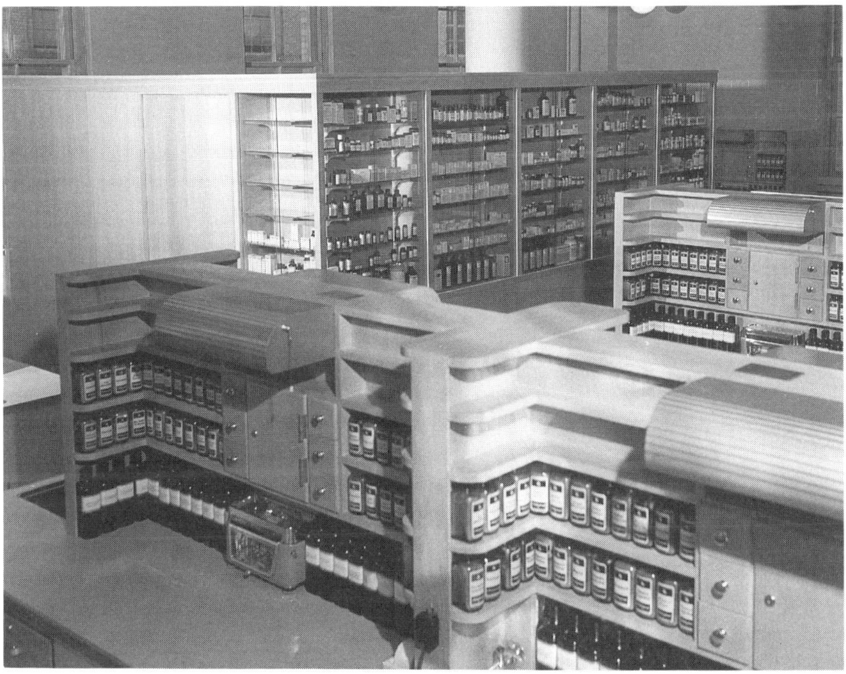

An upgrade of facilities important to undergraduates was this modern dispensing laboratory, opened in 1954 with the help of contributions from Wisconsin pharmacists.

grants from the federal government to individual faculty members for research, and grants to the School from the federal government for the development of its undergraduate programs. The latter funding began in 1970 and lasted about ten years. At the time, there appeared to be a shortage of pharmacists (and of other health professionals) and the federal government provided general operating funds in the form of a "capitation" grant, based on the number of students enrolled. It is not surprising, therefore, that the largest undergraduate enrollments in schools of pharmacy occurred during this period (see *Appendix 4*). Over this ten-year period the funds made available to Wisconsin amounted to as much as 35% of the instructional budget and were still providing about 15% of the budget in 1980, the last year of the "capitation" grant. These grants were used primarily to support a newly developing clinical faculty, and to provide facilities, capital equipment and general supplies to support the expanded student body and the changing curriculum.

As the School's first century ended, extramural research funding (federal and otherwise) was over $1.5 million annually and rising. Such funding had been important throughout most of the century, sought aggressively to do the "extra" things that had to be done. As early as 1894 Kremers was able to obtain fellowship support from the state pharmacists for B.Sc. and M.S. students pursuing some research. C. J. Hunkel and J. L. Mead were the first recipients, receiving $400 and $275, respectively.[34] At the same time a small grant was provided for research on volatile oils by the United States Pharmacopeia.[35] Small but significant gifts of this type helped to provide support for various students and research projects over the ensuing years. Of noteworthy long-term value were the annual $500 fellowships awarded by Fritzsche Brothers Co. from 1917 until World War II.[34]

In 1917, Kremers made the Pharmaceutical Experimental Station the basis for establishing a Wisconsin Pharmaceutical Research Fund. Soliciting individuals and corporations, he established an endowment of over $10,000 by 1926, the principal of which, in part, could be used to support ongoing research[36] By 1982 that fund had grown to over $75,000. In 1958, the 75th year of the School, another special fund designed to provide an endowment for pharmaceutical research was established through the Wisconsin Pharmaceutical Association. Two further examples of generous endowments are a $100,000 loan fund provided by Oscar Rennebohm, and a scholarship fund of $40,000 provided by Mabel Johnson, an early alumna of the School. The receipt of various gifts and bequests by 1982 had accumulated trust funds amounting to about $275,000 for use as student scholarships and loans, and other general purposes.

F. B. Power Pharmaceutical Library

Over its first century the School brought together a pharmaceutical collection unsurpassed by any American university. By 1981 the bound-volume collection housed in the School of Pharmacy Library (including journals) totaled 31,329. In addition there were 121 microfilms, 13,900 microfiches (Iowa Drug Information system), and 412 subscriptions to periodicals. Compared with pharmacy collections elsewhere, Wisconsin's collection probably is most notable for its international outlook and historical depth.

A number of special collections are housed in a historical section of the library, the Kremers Reference Files. Begun early in the century by Kremers, this vertical-file collection, mostly post–1870s material, grew to 710 file drawers, for use by those working in the pharmacohistorical field. In addition, an unknown amount of books and journals dating from 1480 to the 1930s, and later—many thousands of pharmaceutical items—are found in the Memorial Library of the University Library.[37] Moreover, a treasure-trove of pharmaceutical Americana in manuscript form has been accumulating since 1970 in the Archives Division of the State Historical Society of Wisconsin on the Madison campus, under the sponsorship of the American Institute of the History of Pharmacy.

The historical dimension of the collections made UW a center for cultivating pharmacy's history and the obvious site, in 1941, for establishing an American Institute of the History of Pharmacy. Founded at the initiative of Professors Urdang and Kremers, with strong support from Dean Uhl and other faculty, the Institute meanwhile has developed into a unique national agency for the humanistic side of the profession.

The development of this library collection began early in the life of the School, at first primarily by means of personal and corporate donations, and by exchange with other libraries. Even as early as 1900 the collection was claimed to be "one of the best and largest in the country"[38] of its kind. The central library of the University housed most of this collection, while the School, then housed in North Hall, maintained a small collection of duplicate volumes and other materials in its own reading room. Through the consistent efforts of Kremers and later faculty members significant amounts of University resources went into the purchase of important pharmaco-historical books, many of which are now housed in the Department of Special Collections in the Memorial Library.

Throughout the period 1900 to 1950, when the School was housed in North Hall and then in the Chemistry building and was part of the College of Letters and Sciences, a significant effort with very limited resources was made to build up the reading room at the School. In 1927

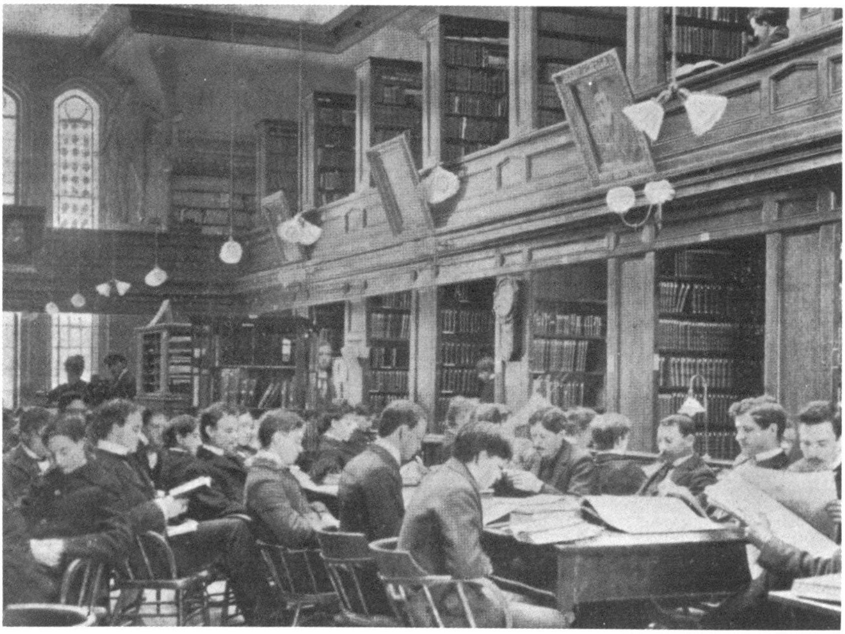

Library collections have been a major resource for all curricular areas in the School since early in the century. At first, pharmacy students searched the literature and studied in the UW General Library (now Music Hall), shown above in 1893. A separate branch library within the School was authorized in 1950, shown below as it looked in the 1970s.

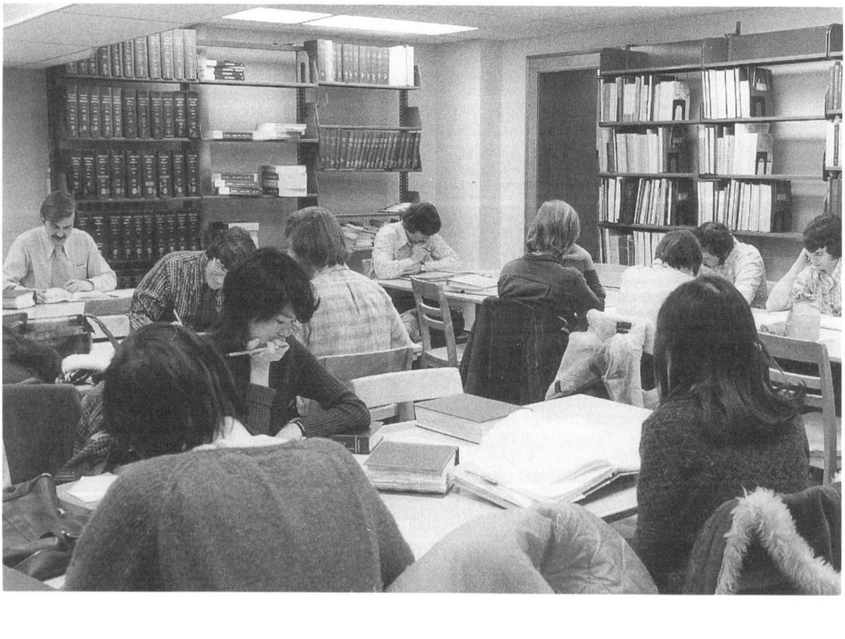

F. B. Power died and left his scientific library to the School of Pharmacy with the stipulation that it be "placed in the building in which pharmacy and pharmaceutical chemistry are taught."[39] The School's entire collection was designated the Frederick B. Power Pharmaceutical Library shortly afterwards, a name retained over the decades. During this period the part of the pharmacy collection that was housed within the School had no professional library services, only receiving minimal attention.

When the School assumed independent status (1950), it housed a collection of 3,550 volumes that became an official branch library of the University Library System. This meant that the budget for personnel and acquisitions was taken over by the Memorial Library. Most of the pharmacy books in the Memorial Library remained there, but were supplemented in subsequent decades mainly as a pharmacohistorical collection.

There have been three professional librarians in charge of the F. B. Power Pharmaceutical Library: James L. Jones, 1950–55; Elsa Reich, 1956–60; and Dolores Nemec, 1961– .

The Library always shared in the housing problems of the School. After becoming an official branch of the UW Library (1950), the Library was better housed and staffed, occupying 3,126 sq. ft. in the west wing. When the Library (combined with the Kremers Reference Files) was moved to the east-wing basement in 1974, its floor space almost doubled. But an outpouring of pharmaceutical literature from publishers soon overcrowded the stacks again—even after a move to the floor above in 1989. Planning for the second century merged the pharmacy collection administratively with the Health Sciences Library, and looked toward eventually combining the collections in a free-standing library building. These library facilities serve as a major source of drug-related information for the State of Wisconsin and beyond.

The Milwaukee Branch

In 1923 the University Board of Regents authorized the Milwaukee Extension Division to offer freshman and sophomore courses for students wishing to complete some of their college education in Milwaukee before going to Madison. In 1947 a department of pharmacy was established in Milwaukee under the direction of Arthur H. Uhl, Director of the School of Pharmacy in Madison. After Max Lemberger, Sr., a prominent Milwaukee pharmacist, served a year as part-time instructor, Dr. Eunice Bonow joined the department on a full-time basis. To accommodate the program, new laboratory facilities were built to teach microbiology and pharmacy preparations, and a small pharmacy library and reading room were established. Students enrolled could complete the first two years of the four-year pharmacy program before moving to Madison.

In 1955 the Milwaukee Extension Division merged with the Wisconsin State College to form the University of Wisconsin–Milwaukee. Five years later, with a new five-year pharmacy curriculum (B.Sc.) in place, it was possible to enroll as a prepharmacy student for two years, apply to the School of Pharmacy and then complete one more year before going to Madison. For students living in the Milwaukee area this was a convenient arrangement and the program attracted a large student group. In 1960 a second faculty member was employed, and the program continued at this level until 1973 when, apparently for economic reasons, it was decided to offer only the prepharmacy portion of the program.

Student Enrollments: Quality vs Quantity

It has often been said that a great educational institution exists when a combination exists of quality teachers, motivated and bright students, and the resources to support the academic environment required. A dilemma arises in reconciling the need for resources with the danger of lowering standards of admission and instruction to maintain enrollments at a level required to justify resources.

From its inception the School of Pharmacy has had to face a number of issues that centered on enrollments and the quality of education. In the early years enrollments were low, whereas in later years enrollments rose dramatically. It is of interest to briefly explore this issue because it tells us something about the way this school has operated and the character of its leadership and faculty during those times.

In the late nineteenth century formal education was not legally required to practice pharmacy in any state, and competition for students among independent schools was keen. As head of one of only two pharmacy programs integrated with and supported by a state university, Power avowed "the higher aim of securing earnest, capable and industrious students with the conviction that *quality* should be a much more important consideration than quantity."[12] Enrollment figures for the period of Power's tenure exhibited a slow but steady growth and there was a correspondingly modest increase in the resources made available to the School.

From enrollment figures for the period soon after Power left, it is clear that a number of significant changes took place. First of all we see that initially (1892) 2 out of 64 students opted for the new four-year B.Sc. program, although the number increased during the next few years. Of greater significance, a large number of students opted to take the three-year program rather than the two-year program, even though both led to the Ph.G. diploma. It is clear from what we have already learned about Edward Kremers that, upon taking over the position of leadership, he was intent on raising the level of instruction and the standards for admission and graduation. Whereas Power had been sensitive to the concerns of pharmacy practitioners and took a more evolutionary approach to meet his objectives, Kremers had his goals clearly in mind and had a desire to reach them as soon as possible. It is not surprising, therefore, that soon after he took over and put his plans into effect total enrollments showed a significant decline and did not rise appreciably until after World War I.

It is apparent from enrollment figures, however, that the issue of the curriculum not being practical enough[40] (see Chapter 3) was not the sole factor in the lack of growth in enrollment. Rather, much can be attributed to the rigor of the program and the personality of its leader. That concern continued is seen in some of the papers of University President Charles Adams.[41] In various communications to the Board of Regents in 1898 to 1900, Adams expressed great concern about the lack of growth in the School of Pharmacy. He raised questions about the high standards of the program and asked whether these were higher than "the market could bear." He was concerned to learn that druggists were sending students elsewhere and sought their opinion by sending out a letter to 80 "of the most prominent pharmacists in the State." Of the 50 replies about 30 were negative, leading Adams to conclude that the course is too theoretical and not practical enough, possibly because it was founded on "German ideals" entirely different from those which "prevail in this country." Attention was drawn to the fact that not a single practicing pharmacist was on the instructional staff, that the Director was not popular with pharmacists, and that a new school of pharmacy in Milwaukee was taking away all students from Milwaukee who might ordinarily have come to study in Madison. He went so far as to suggest that Kremers should resign, but when Kremers offered to so do, his resignation was not accepted. The matter appears to have been dropped in 1900 with Adams' illness and with some firm support for Kremers from Dean Birge of the College of Letters and Sciences.[42]

Attention is drawn to these incidents to stress the normal concern of University administrations for enrollment growth and the often conflicting dedication of the early leaders of this school to the promotion of quality rather than quantity. Although practical education was perceived by Kremers to be important, he would not sacrifice the fundamental scientific components when support for a chair in practical pharmacy was not forthcoming. He stated on one occasion that if he could not provide quality practical training, he would not do it at all.[40] Although low enrollments contributed to a lack of strong budgetary support in succeeding years, there is no evidence that standards were knowingly lowered as a way of circumventing the issue.

The years following World War II brought an extraordinary number of students, relative to earlier years, requiring temporary teaching quarters for a few years, greatly taxing an understaffed faculty in the School of Pharmacy. This problem was somewhat relieved by the new facilities made available in 1955. Pressure of high enrollments continued to build, however, as college enrollments in general swelled during the 1960s and 1970s. Incoming classes grew to nearly 200 by 1972, encouraged by a period of demand for pharmacists and by federal "capitation" grants that stipulated acceptance of more students, as mentioned earlier. The exceptionally large incoming classes continued until about 1979.

A few years earlier there had been a significant shortage of pharmacists; now the much larger graduating classes led many pharmacists to feel that student enrollments were leading to an oversupply of pharmacists in Wisconsin. The University was accused by many pharmacists of accepting large numbers of students for budgetary reasons only. The University administration's position centered on the issue of supply and demand,[43] maintaining that as long as the applicant pool was bringing in qualified students, and the School had facilities and resources to handle them, it was their responsibility to keep the doors open. It was felt that no school, no professional group should be put in the position of determining the number of individuals entering a particular profession. Then, from 1979 to 1982, the School experienced about a 47% drop in entering-class enrollment, before leveling off. Similar trends were seen nationally without any special effort from the schools of pharmacy to curtail enrollments.[44]

Relations with Pharmacists of the State

The history of the University of Wisconsin School of Pharmacy involves a close relationship between the School and the pharmacists of the state, primarily through the Wisconsin Pharmaceutical Association. References have been made, here and elsewhere, to the role played by the Association in the founding of the School, and its continual involvement in seeking for the School independent status, resources and new facilities. On the other hand, the School faculty and administration have taken an equally active interest in the Association and other professional activities in this state by sponsoring continuing education programs, attending Association meetings and serving on various organizational committees. Two of the Directors, Kremers and Uhl, for example, served as presidents of WPhA. Associate Dean Busse for many years was active in assisting the State Board in the development of a meaningful internship program for Wisconsin[45] and several faculty members have served on the tripartite Internship Board. Both constituencies, the School and the profession, have served as valued resources for each other over the years.

From the beginning, the formal linkages between the School and WPhA were strongly developed. Right after the founding in 1883 a WPhA School of Pharmacy Committee was formed and at Professor Power's request they were invited to come to the School and see for themselves what the various students were doing and actually examine them. During the first years only a few Committee members came on such visits; so in 1887, with the concurrence of Power, the WPhA decided that the entire State Board should function as the liaison Committee, and come to the School each year and administer the licensing examination to the graduates.[46]

During those early years, the School of Pharmacy Committee often presented a report, but more often Power and, later, Kremers would be present at Annual Meetings of the WPhA to review the year's activities at the School, a practice continued to the present day.

Kremers used this opportunity, particularly during the period of 1902 to 1911, to express concern about what he saw as the indifference of the average pharmacist to the School, contrasting this indifference with the active support that the schools of agriculture and engineering were receiving from their constituencies.[47] As early as 1904 he asked that a visiting committee be appointed, saying, "Might it not be proper and well for this Association to appoint a committee to visit the University and to report back to this Association such matters as in the opinion of its members ought to receive attention of this organization?"[48]

A resolution to form a visiting committee was approved at the 1908 Annual Meeting, but there is no evidence that it functioned to his satisfaction, if at all, since Kremers continued to express concern about the lack of pharmacists' interest during the rest of his tenure as Director. Strong interactions between the School and the Association continued to occur, but given Kremers' personality and style, many pharmacists probably found it hard to respond to his urgings for more financial and political support in attaining the goals of the School. There was no lack of respect for Kremers—an educator of exceptional breadth and depth, even judged by an international standard. Yet, up to the time of Kremers' retirement in 1935, except for some attempts at getting a new building, the Association had generated few sustained efforts toward assisting the School.

Kremers' successor, Arthur H. Uhl, recognized the important role the School could play in promoting the profession and realized that the School needed the support of the pharmacists in such areas as recruitment of students, financial aid, and obtaining facilities and independent status. He clearly made an extraordinary effort to interact with the pharmacists of Wisconsin, both personally and through faculty participation—through continuing education programs, representation at district and local association meetings, joint committees on internship, development of a branch in Milwaukee, and in general, high visibility in professional affairs. Not all pharmacists agreed with everything the School was doing, but an exceptionally friendly relationship developed.

In view of this stronger identification of pharmacists with the School, it is, perhaps, not surprising that in 1967 and 1968 many practitioners actively expressed opposition to the appointment as dean of David Perlman, a distinguished pharmaceutical scientist who had joined the

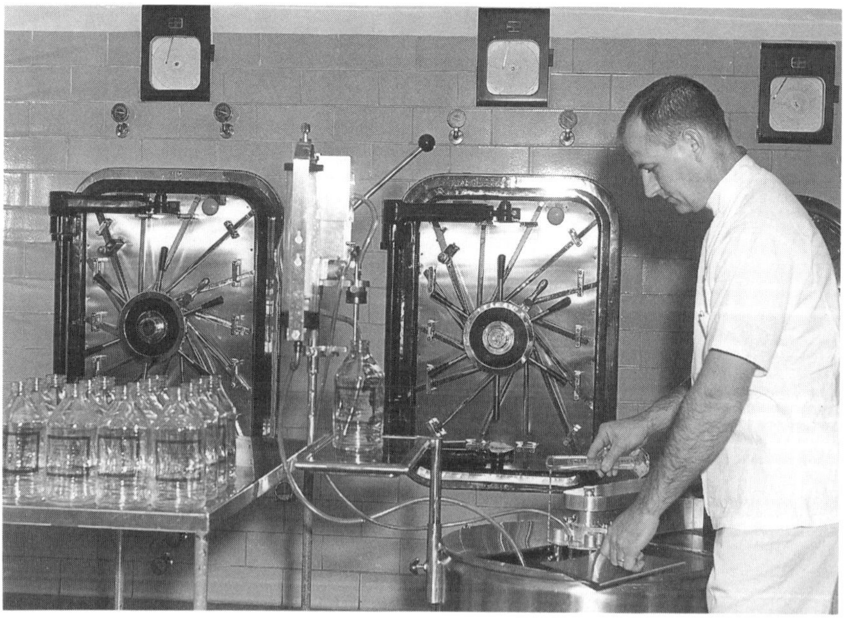

Resources for teaching hospital pharmacy improved greatly after the new University Hospital opened in 1977, and its wards became increasingly important for clerkships as clinical pharmacy developed as a practice orientation.

School of Pharmacy faculty one year earlier. The reasons generally given for this opposition were his lack of professional pharmaceutical education and the short period he had been in pharmaceutical education. There was concern in the state association and among individual practitioners that the commitment of the School to professional pharmacy might not be adequately addressed. So strong were the charges and countercharges that in 1968, after appointing Dr. Perlman as dean, the Board of Regents met at the urging of the Wisconsin Pharmaceutical Association to reconsider their earlier action.[49] Their earlier action, however, was reaffirmed and Perlman became dean on July 1, 1968 (see *Appendix 1*). This single event had a far-reaching effect on the attitudes toward the School and University among pharmacy alumni all around the state and country.

Despite extraordinary efforts by Dean Perlman to demonstrate his interest and concern for professional matters, he never received the widespread support from the alumni and pharmacists that his predecessor had had. Would this have happened at another school in a similar situation? Or was the relationship between the School and profession, or between the conflicting individuals and ideas, so peculiar to Wisconsin that it triggered an unprecedented attempt to overthrow the University's appointment of a dean? In any event it is remembered as a low point in the life of pharmacy in Wisconsin.

Entering the second century with new leadership in both the School and Association, with new issues vying for attention, the deanship controversy cooled and relationships improved. Turning to face what seemed unprecedented professional change, Wisconsin practitioners resumed a traditional, if uneasy, alliance with the faculty in Madison.

Continuing Education

From its earliest years, the University of Wisconsin committed itself to serving the people of Wisconsin through continuing education and related activities.[50] This aspect of its role, which came to be known as the "Wisconsin Idea," brought recognition and honor to the University and reaped great benefits for the citizens who participated in the many continuing education programs offered over the decades. It was natural that the School of Pharmacy would be an active participant in the "Wisconsin Idea," and, indeed, it became a leader in showing the way toward continuing education in pharmacy nationally.

As early as 1900, the Board of Regents, at the request of Edward Kremers, authorized a special summer session for the School of Pharmacy.

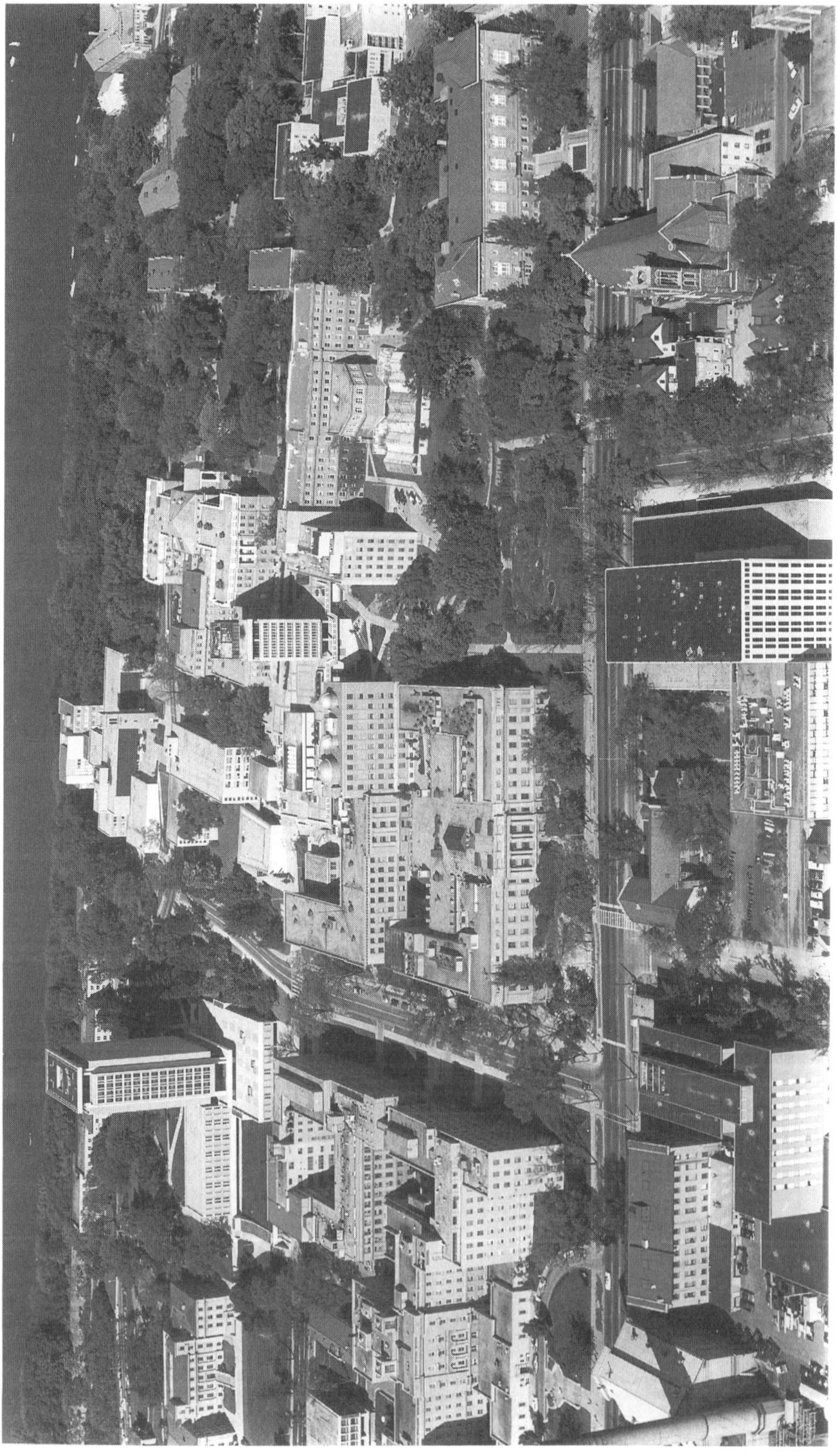

This was a six-week session of laboratory courses intended for apprentices and clerks who could not take the regular University courses. Unfortunately, it attracted only five students in 1900 and two students in 1901, so the program was not repeated again until 1914, when again it had only limited success. In 1909 there was another attempt to provide basic instruction—which Kremers felt was so important for those unable to attend the University—through special lectures in chemistry and pharmaceutical chemistry, and this was somewhat more successful. Through the University Extension Division 13 correspondence courses in the pharmaceutical sciences were also developed, for students entering the University as well as for pharmacists wishing to obtain some continuing education. Such correspondence courses, which continued to be offered well into the 1920s, were rigorous. For example, in 1924 the percentage of those not completing the course was as high as 85%.[51]

In 1909, special postgraduate courses in business administration also were offered. The announcement said, ". . . while the college student or clerk preparing for the State Board Examination is kept more than busy with his professional studies, the pharmaceutical graduate and the registered pharmacist may well give attention to this important subject. The courses offered comprise something more than mere instruction in the writing of business papers."[52]

Such a statement reflected the feeling of Kremers that it was the job of the School to provide the fundamental basis for pharmaceutical practice, including the business aspects of the profession.

In 1936, the federal government, through the George Deen Act,[53] began to provide aid to states for the vocational training of "distributive workers." Wisconsin became one of the few states to take advantage of this act for pharmacy when, in 1937, the Wisconsin State Board of Pharmacy, the Wisconsin Pharmaceutical Association and the Wisconsin State Board of Vocational and Adult Education initiated a program directed toward community pharmacists.

In the years 1937–40, a "circuit instructor," pharmacist Edwin J. Boberg, traveled to eight cities in Wisconsin, and at the vocational schools located there he offered biweekly evening courses in practical matters associated with the operation of a retail shop. These were not thought of

This aerial photograph, looking toward the Lake Mendota shore, shows the ideal central location of the building at Charter Street and University Avenue (at center, with pillars), which the School of Pharmacy shared with Chemistry from 1905 and with Physics from 1967. But facilities of the School had become outgrown and outmoded by the end of its first century.

as college-level subjects, so the School of Pharmacy did not provide any expertise or input, although the Director of the School, A. H. Uhl, did support the idea of such a program.[54]

It was not until the late 1950s that the School of Pharmacy again moved aggressively in developing a presence around the state through continuing education. About 1950 Louis W. Busse assumed responsibility for developing continuing education pharmacy programs together with the University Extension Division. In 1951, William S. Apple, then studying for a doctorate in pharmacy administration, was appointed to coordinate extension programs in Pharmacy on a part-time basis, and this gave great impetus to a number of activities.

This period led to the establishment of two important annual programs, which continue to be offered, the Fall Pharmacy Institute and the Spring Pharmacy Management Institute. The Fall Institute, jointly sponsored with WPhA, brought over a hundred pharmacists to Madison for three days of teaching programs and alumni activities. Typical of the earlier programs was the one in 1951, which provided lecture and laboratory instruction on the uses of dermatological preparations, as well a program which addressed contemporary issues in pharmacy, such as "Must Wisconsin Physicians Dispense?". From the 1970s, the programs focussed more frequently on disease states and the use of therapeutic agents for their treatment.

The Spring Management Institute, on the other hand, devoted itself exclusively to the economic and management aspects of community and hospital pharmacies. A concurrent annual activity was a High School Counselling Program, which provided high school students from around the state an opportunity to visit the School and to learn about career opportunities in pharmacy. Each of the high school students attending was the guest of a hometown pharmacist.

In 1956 a formal arrangement between the School of Pharmacy and the Extension Division created a department of pharmacy within Extension, known as Extension Services in Pharmacy. Associate Dean Busse was appointed director (with a 25% appointment in Extension) and Richard S. Strommen became the full-time extension coordinator. In 1959 the program made its first move to meet the continuing education needs of industrial pharmacists by establishing a week-long teaching conference in Land O' Lakes, Wisconsin (see p. 153). The Land O' Lakes conferences were designed to provide basic instruction in the underlying principles for work in drug product research and development. Offered in June each year, the conference was planned and executed by the School faculty and experts from the pharmaceutical industry. The relaxed atmosphere of the Wisconsin woods was very conducive for individual and small-group interactions. This success led in 1962 to the establishment of the "August Land O' Lakes Conferences" on pharmaceutical analysis and quality control. Both series of conferences have maintained their popularity and usefulness.

In 1964, Dr. William Blockstein assumed the position of full-time extension coordinator, while in 1965 Dr. August P. Lemberger assumed Busse's position as director. For the next few years, particularly with the faculty appointment of Dr. Jens T. Carstensen, an established industrial scientist, a concerted and successful effort was made to develop a series of industrial "short courses." Such courses, taught intensively for one week, brought 15 to 20 students together in lecture and laboratory sessions, dealing with such topics as disperse systems, solid dosage forms, pharmacokinetics and biopharmaceutics. This was expanded to include courses in statistical methods and pharmacology for chemists. With the increased regulation of the pharmaceutical industry by the Food and Drug Administration, an annual program on regulatory affairs also proved quite successful.

In the area of professional pharmacy, UW continuing education, in the late 1960s, established two programs with significant impact. Through the use of a statewide telephone network, it was possible in 1966 to provide live lectures to numerous classrooms around the state where pharmacists could gather for a few hours each week for a full semester course. Two-way hookups allowed questions to be asked of the lecturer, and written prepared notes provided material to augment the lectures. An average of about 500 pharmacists and other health professionals attended these courses each year. Another program, started in 1972 with "seed funds" from capitation funds of the School of Pharmacy, involved the preparation by faculty of 8 to 11 audio-cassettes on a single topic, with accompanying written material for self-paced instruction. During just the first decade of the program, 24 such series were prepared, and a total of about 120,000 copies were distributed nationwide.

In 1969 with the merger of all state higher educational institutions into the University of Wisconsin System, extension activities statewide were brought together into a separate, university-level, administrative unit, called the University of Wisconsin–Extension. Blockstein assumed the chairmanship of the unit of Health Sciences and Dr. Melvin Weinswig was brought in as chairman of the pharmacy department within this new unit and given a 25% appointment on the School of Pharmacy faculty. The program grew to include four full-time professional positions, administratively separate, but each holding some type of appointment in the School. The department, now administered by the School of Pharmacy, continues to be housed in School facilities and programs are cooperatively sponsored and planned.

Notes and References

1. Merle Curti and Vernon Carstensen, *The University of Wisconsin, A History, 1848–1925*, II (Madison, 1949), 29.
2. School of Pharmacy Committee, "The School of Pharmacy," *Proc. WPhA 1916*, 109 f.
3. Curti and Carstensen, (n. 1) II, 1949, 30.
4. *Report of the American Council on Pharmaceutical Education, 1949*, ms, KRF, C31(a) I:Wis.
5. A. H. Uhl papers, KRF, A2, (1949).
6. Ibid.
7. Anon., "Separate School of Pharmacy," *Wis. Drugg*. 17 (1949): No. 10, p.7.
8. *Proceedings, Conference on Pharmacy Medicine and Nursing, University of Michigan* (Ann Arbor, 1967).
9. D. Perlman, Dean, to E. Young, Chancellor, March 15, 1971, Papers of H. Edwin Young, Archives.
10. D. Perlman, Dean, personal comments to George Zografi, 1971.
11. *Badger Pharmacist* (Madison, 1900), 115.
12. F. B. Power, "The Department of Pharmacy," *Proc. WPhA*, 1891, 11.
13. E. Kremers, *Proc WPhA., 1925*, 68. A revealing and critical address to practitioners.
14. Fr. Hoffmann, "Die Pharmacie-Schule, Universität des Staates Wisconsin," *Pharmaceutische Rundschau*, 8 (1890): 175–182.
15. E. Kremers to G. C. Sellery, Dean, 1926, KRF, C31(a) I: Wis.
16. E. Kremers, "The School of Pharmacy," *Proc. WPhA, 1896*, 42.
17. A. H. Uhl, personal comments to George Zografi, 1975.
18. Glenn Sonnedecker and Louis W. Busse, personal interview by George Zografi, 1981.
19. David Perlman, personal comments to George Zografi, 1975.
20. *American Council on Pharmaceutical Education Accreditation Manual, 1975.*
21. *Proc.WPhA, 1900*, 35.
22. Kremers, (n. 16), 43.
23. "School of Pharmacy Committee Report," ibid., 1924, 167.
24. Oscar Rennebohm, *WPhA Proc. 1927*, 52.
25. "School of Pharmacy Committee Report," ibid., 1930, 117.
26. S. R. Chechik, "Report of the New School of Pharmacy Building Committee,"

Wis. Drugg. 13 (1945): No. 11, p. 40.

27. L. F. Madland, *Wis. Drugg*. 15 (1947) : No. 4, P. 28.
28. A. H. Uhl papers, 1949, KRF, C31(a)I Wis.
29. Ibid.
30. "Report of Committee on School of Pharmacy," *Proc. WPhA 1883*, 40 and 43.
31. University of Wisconsin Budget Books, 1895–96, Archives.
32. "Report of Committee on School of Pharmacy," *Proc. WPhA 1913*, 24.
33. Edward Kremers, "Report on the School of Pharmacy," *Proc WPhA 1898*, 28.
34. Fellowship file, 1920–29, KRF, C31(a)I: Wis.
35. *School of Pharmacy. . . Bulletin*, 1895–96, 228.
36. Anon., "The Wisconsin School of Pharmacy," *Wis. Drugg*. 7 (1939): No. 8, pp. 8–10.
37. To obtain an impression of the rarities available, see John Neu, *Chemical, Medical and Pharmaceutical Books Printed Belore 1800; In the Collections of the University of Wisconsin Libraries* (Madison, 1965), 280 pp., and G.J. Higby and E.C. Stroud, "Pharmaco-Historical Resources in Madison, Wisconsin, "*Pharm. Hist*. 30 (1988): 33–36, 99–102, 157–162, 195–198 (& collated reprint).
38. *Badger Pharmacist* (n. 11), 138.
39. Oscar Rennebohm, [report on School], *Proc. WPhA 1927*, 50.
40. Edward Kremers, to President Charles Adams, April 16, 1895, KRF, C31(a) I: Wis.
41. Charles Adams, report to Board of Regents, University of Wisconsin, Jan. 1899, 483.
42. Ibid., Feb. 1900, 575 and 590.
43. George Zografi, Dean [report to WPhA], ms., 1976.
44. John F. Schlegel, "Current Perceptions and Facts Concerning Manpower Needs," *NABP/AACP District Four, Proc. 1981*, 20. As the School began its second century, entering-class enrollments varied (1984–94) within a rather narrow range of 106 to 125.
45. Louis W. Busse, "Pharmacy Internship Training," *J. Am. Pharm. Assoc*. (Pract. Pharm. Ed.), 18 (1957): 612.
46. *Proc.WPhA, 1887*, 46.
47. Ibid., 1902, 45.
48. Ibid., 1904, 57.
49. President William Sewell, letter to "Wisconsin Pharmacists," June 5, 1968, Archives.
50. Curti and Carstensen (n. 1), II, 1949, 549.
51. Robert A. Buerki, "Historical Development of Continuing Pharmaceutical Education in American Universities," unpublished Ph.D. thesis, Ohio State University, 1972, 114.
52. Ibid., 95.
53. Ibid., 258.
54. Ibid., 186.

CHAPTER 3

The Curriculum

BY GLENN SONNEDECKER

A CURRICULUM to a faculty is like a road map to a traveller. As with any map, a curriculum needs periodic updating, if students are to reach their destination. As a work in progress it occasionally entails a detour, especially if academic decision-making is complicated by university fiscal restraints, or by the different biases of scientist and practitioner, or by the vagaries of an approval process that extends beyond a particular school or department, or by the importuning of special-interest groups among alumni. Such cross-currents can be sensed on occasion when the evolution of the UW pharmacy curriculum is examined, but their influence has not been fully interpreted here, given the sparse records and the limited space available.

In the Classroom, 1884–85

In the early years of the century curriculum-building was a simpler process, when Frederick Power constituted a one-man pharmacy department and taught all the pharmaceutical subjects himself. What it must have been like to sit in his classes can be glimpsed through the syllabi for 1884–85 that he jotted down in the back of an old notebook. In the front of this historic document are the course notes that Power took years before as a student at the Philadelphia College of Pharmacy.

In Power's class at Wisconsin for "Practical Pharmacy and Pharmaceutical Chemistry" a student first heard three lectures on metrology and apparatus. This was followed by seven periods on the processes for making medicaments (e.g., decoctions, fluidextracts, and medicated waters). The remaining forty-one periods were devoted to medicinal chemicals (e.g., inorganic and organic acids, the relevant salts of elements such as the halogens, potassium and sodium, antimony, sulfur and mercury, and the "officinal spirits" such as medicinal wines, chloroform and chloral, and ethers). Pharmaceutical necessities discussed included honey, grape sugars and malt.

In the "Materia Medica" course a student studied the natural history and uses of about 260 botanical drugs, beginning with Ergot, Ustillago, Chondrus crispus, and Fucus vesiculosus, and ending forty-nine lectures later with Tamarind, Acacia and Catechu. By the 1880s only six substances of animal origin any longer merited attention: Cantharis, Moschus, Castoreum, Coccus, Ichthyocolla and Gelatin.

When we examine Power's syllabus for the "Pharmaceutical Laboratory" in the second year of the curriculum, it seems demanding for its time. Medicinal chemicals were prepared by the student, such as potassium acetate and iron citrate. Crude drugs were assayed, such as opium and cinchona bark. Practice in typical processes included percolation

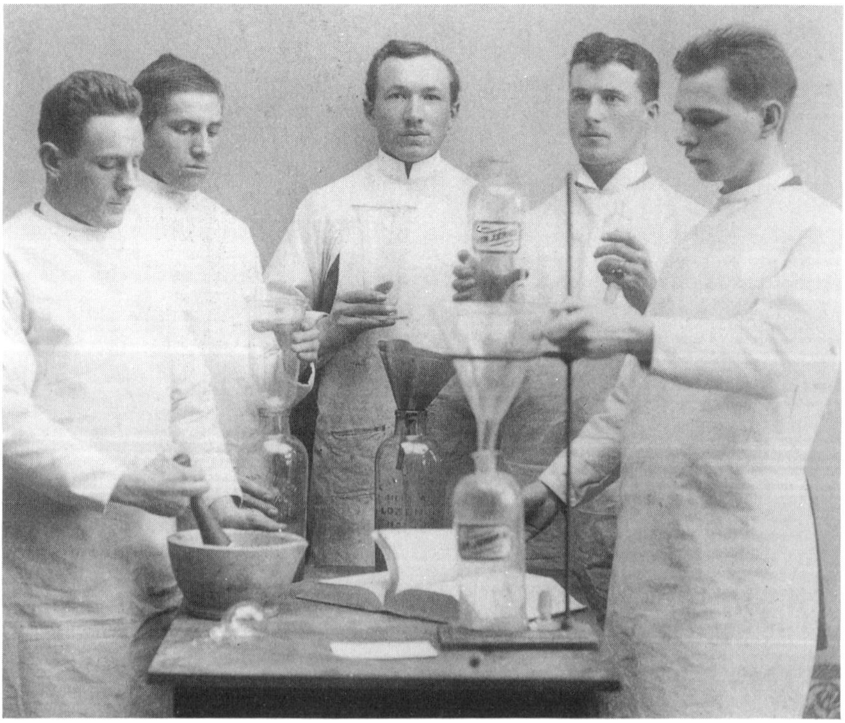

Five students in the course on "practical pharmacy," 1888–89, pretend work to accommodate a photographer. The only student identified, Rudolph Wiese of Milwaukee (far right), had selected the theme "Liniments of the National Formulary" for the thesis required in the two-year curriculum.

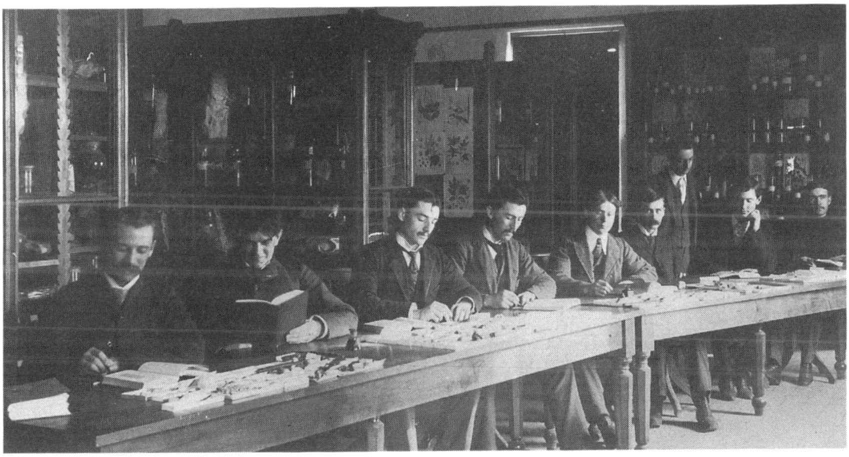

Students in the 1890s are learning to identify each crude drug by sight, and are studying its production and processing, its pharmaceutical and therapeutic properties. The traditional study of materia medica remained important into the 1930s.

(wild cherry bark), crystallization (sodium and potassium tartrate), emulsification (castor oil), plasters (e.g., adhesive) and suppositories (belladonna). Altogether there were twenty laboratory periods during the semester (September 23 to December 10, 1884), including three periods for faculty demonstrations.[1]

Wisconsin's first pharmacy students were expected to work in the laboratory "four hours daily" throughout the second year of the curriculum, one recalled, but "were permitted to work all day long in the laboratory if we so desired."[2] A student capable of undertaking extended work was urged to do so during the first year, "as opportunity will thereby be afforded during the Senior year for more advanced study of analytical chemistry and for original research and investigation."[3] Pharmacy thus became one of the first departments on the campus to emphasize research. The status of applied science in the wider mission of land-grant universities readily supported a laboratory orientation in the pharmacy curriculum. The independent pharmacy colleges introduced laboratory science more hesitantly because of the high cost and the low support among their practitioner-sponsors. In a university, intellectual standards of the institution at large only partially insulated a pharmacy curriculum from the influence of practitioners. They argued for a practical training more clearly within the ability of their apprentices, a majority of whom had not graduated from high school.[4]

The conceptual difference was put in perspective by Edward Kremers when he later observed: "There are two distinct tendencies which manifest themselves to the student of pharmaceutical education in this country; the first found its highest expression in the establishment of the older (independent) colleges of pharmacy, the outcome of the ambitions and ideals of the apothecary guilds of several of our larger eastern cities, a product of English ideas, traditions and influences; the second found its expression in the establishment of departments and schools of pharmacy at our state universities at a time when American educational ideas were undergoing marked changes due to the influence of German educational ideas and methods."[5]

A Controversial Innovator

When Power was lured away by industry he was succeeded in 1892 by Kremers, a Wisconsin pharmacist who had experienced a rigorous apprenticeship with an immigrant German pharmacist and earned a German Ph.D. degree (see p. 171). This young instructor returned from Germany fired up for curricular reform.[6] If Power had seemed reluctant to match the bold curricular approach of Albert Prescott at the University of Michigan, the new director of the program, age 27, showed no such reluctance. Kremers promptly proclaimed "the good fortune of the School of Pharmacy to be able to announce a decided improvement in its course." In the fall 1892 he added an optional four-year curriculum (see *Appendix 3*). It was a move unprecedented in American pharmacy. The President of the

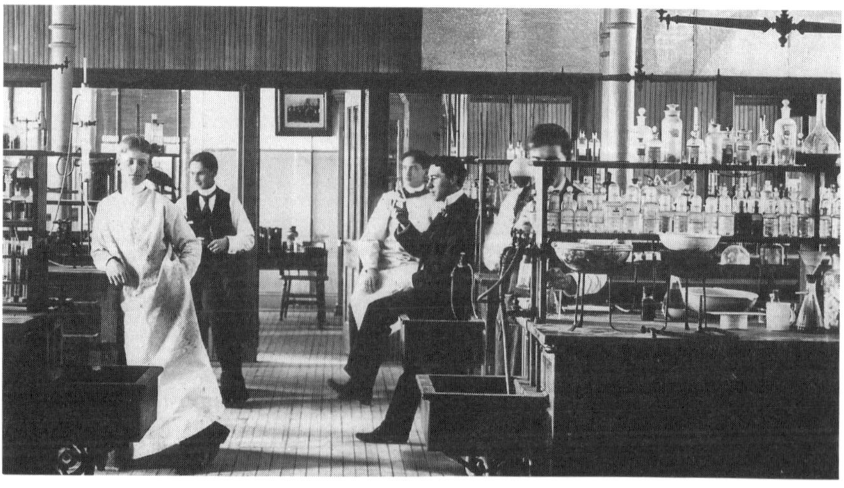

Students in this "pharm chem lab" of the 1890s had fulfilled the School's prerequisite of a year's study of general chemistry.

University had some misgivings about this innovation and asked Kremers how many students he expected to have in the new program. He reportedly replied: "Mr. President, I am not concerned with numbers, but with an ideal."[7]

Kremers thus established the principle of offering education in pharmacy on par with standard baccalaureate programs in the University. But only a minority of the students, given a choice, would choose the new four-year curriculum. For example, there were four times as many two- and three-year graduates as four-year graduates during the first decade that the B.Sc. in Pharmacy was being conferred.

Unlike the required two-year curriculum—which had one year of high school (or equivalent) as a prerequisite—the optional four-year sequence required high-school graduation (or equivalent). Moreover, students in both curricula henceforth studied during the full academic year. Previously, pharmacy courses had been only about two-thirds as long as the University's standard year. Kremers assured recruits that "the object of the course has been and still is to lay as thorough a scientific foundation as time and means will permit for the pursuit of the profession of pharmacy. . . .The methods of work differ in no essential from those adopted for the other scientific departments [of the University] . . . ."[8]

The department thus gave notice that pharmacy intended to become a full-fledged member of the University community. However, practitioners throughout the state (9 out of 10 never having graduated from any university program) were getting more than bargained for when they engineered the founding of the department about a decade earlier. At the Wisconsin Pharmaceutical Association (WPhA) meeting in 1893, John A. Dadd, a respected Milwaukee pharmacist, spoke critically about apprentices being "kept at studies which do not fit them for the practical duties of a pharmacist," claiming "that there is a great dissatisfaction expressed with the manner in which the School of Pharmacy of the University is conducted since the departure of Professor Power. . . ." Kremers responded that apprentices coming to the University were "not sufficiently prepared," as evidenced in the drop from 64 to 46 students during the course of the year. "The druggists of the state are invited," said Kremers, "to give more care and consideration to the selection of their apprentices. . . ." Rarely one to sugarcoat a pill, he added that the UW's curriculum "is particularly strong on the theoretical side" and that a course in physics was being added to the two-year curriculum, and laboratory work with medicinal plants would be required, including botanical field trips.[9] Field trips also were scheduled to several Milwaukee chemical manufactories.

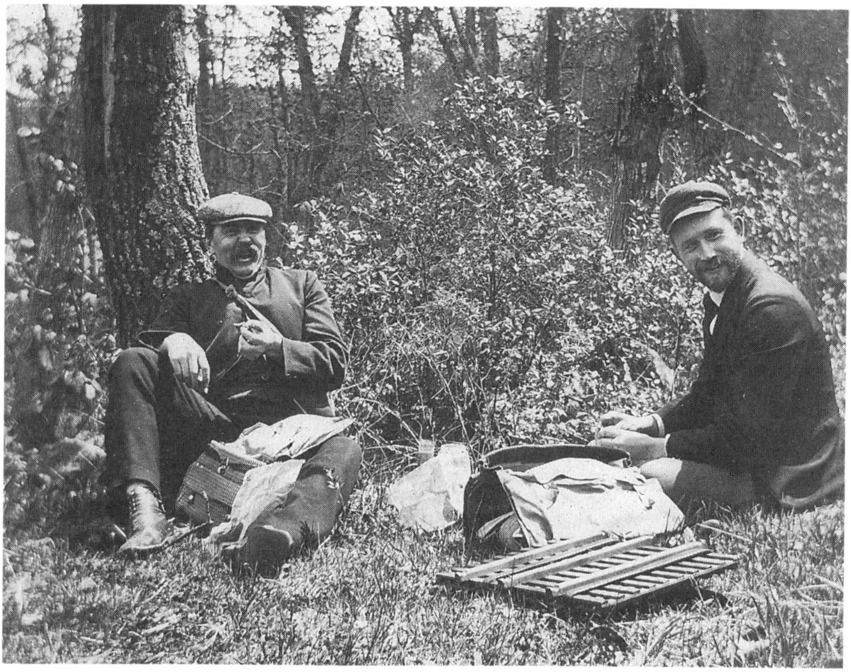

Botanizing excursions to learn about Wisconsin's medicinal plants were a Saturday feature of one of the courses in pharmaceutical botany about 1900. The "Drug Cabinet" at this time contained some five thousand specimens of crude drugs.

Kremers' spirited response was only the first of a series of skirmishes that lay ahead between the scientific idealist at UW and his practical-minded constituents.

Already in the following year controversy erupted when Kremers recommended to the WPhA that the graduation requirement of four years' apprenticeship be deleted. A special committee agreed with Kremers, especially since apprenticeship could be continued as a requirement for licensure by the State Board of Pharmacy. Sensing a fait accompli, the Association tabled the issue, "as the [UW] Regents had [already] made the changes and the Association had no voice in the matter. . . ."[10] It was a harbinger that the Association's paternal influence on the University was waning.

Despite continued development of the School of Pharmacy, no academic education was legally required to practice pharmacy in Wisconsin, although passing a state licensure examination had been required since 1882—after an initial registration by "grandfathering" the existing practitioners. To save time and money in preparing for the examination, apprentices often preferred one of the proprietary "cram schools," including at

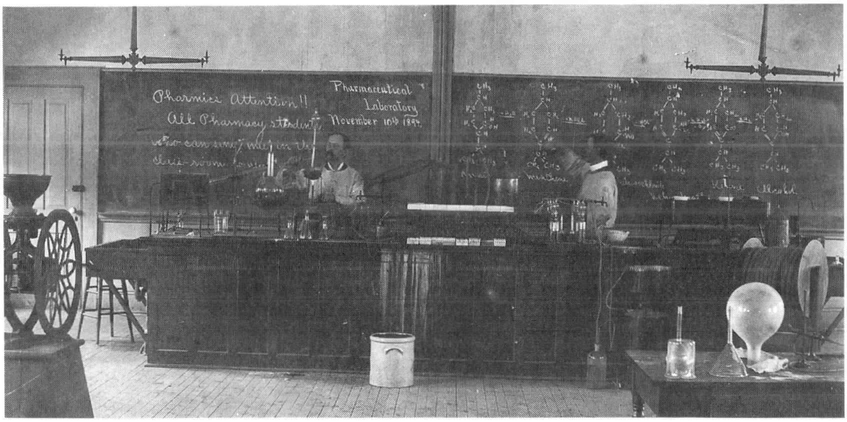

Organic reactions being written on the blackboard in 1894 are not unlike those dreaded by countless generations of pharmacy students. The blackboard also admonishes, "All pharmacy students who can sing meet in the classroom tonight . . . ."

least two in Wisconsin.[11] The demand for a University education was further undercut by the ready availability of certificates as "Assistant Pharmacists" (322 in 1895), who were employed much like licensed Pharmacists.[12]

A further damper on standards stemmed from keen competition among schools of pharmacy around the turn of the century. The Wisconsin program felt the effect of two Chicago schools, which lured students with a more elementary curriculum and a stint of big-city life, and the effect of a pharmacy department (f.1899) in the Milwaukee Medical College, whose pharmacy curriculum was "modeled more after those of the Chicago colleges than those of the University."[13]

In 1905 a New York State law became effective that influenced pharmaceutical education nationally. It required a high-school diploma or equivalent and graduation from at least a two-year pharmacy curriculum to qualify for licensure examination. Moreover, the curriculum had to meet specifications laid out in the *Pharmaceutical Syllabus* (1910, 146 pp.).[14]

At Wisconsin, most students continued to enroll in a modified two-year curriculum (see *Appendix 3*, p. 189). Kremers himself held an unshakable faith in the advantage to practicing pharmacists of having the better scientific foundation afforded by the four-year curriculum. Additionally, the B.Sc. degree opened to ambitious students the possibility of earning advanced degrees (see Chapter 5). Wisconsin set the example for five other university schools of pharmacy that adopted an optional four-year curriculum by the turn of the century, but the average Wisconsin practitioner apparently remained unenthusiastic about the UW initiative.

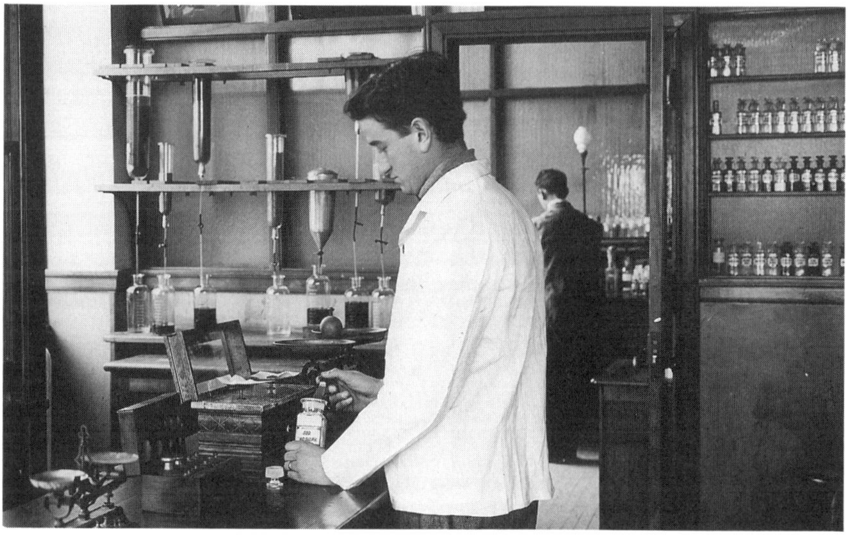

Students learned the preparation of dosage forms, from crude drugs to finished product. For example, a rack of small-scale percolators is featured in this scene from early in the century.

"Instead of incorporating into our annual proceedings the usual report that the School of Pharmacy is doing as well as may be expected," the Committee on School of Pharmacy told WPhA members in 1923, ". . . let us recognize that there is a certain amount of dissension which prevents the association and the school from working together in harmony for the common good. . . . Dr. Kremers is held up as being too theoretical, too visionary, not practical."[15]

The Three-Year Curriculum

To Kremers it would have seemed a timely advantage to pharmacy and to Wisconsin patients if all pharmacy graduates earned the University's standard Bachelor's degree. Instead, the School established a three-year curriculum as the minimum program, starting with admissions in the fall of 1925. The School thus complied with a new requirement for eligibility to membership in the American Conference of Pharmaceutical Faculties.[16] Further delay would have jeopardized the right of future graduates to reciprocate their license when moving to another state.

In announcing the three-year curriculum (see *Appendix 3*, p. 191) the School indicated that the course "has been carefully planned to accommodate those students who are unable to remain four years at the University, as well as to meet the advancing requirements of pharmaceutical education," and noted that Ph.G. graduates "may return to the University and complete the requirements of the four-year course in one year."[17] A three-year program was not entirely new to Wisconsin, having been a third curricular option offered to students between 1894 and 1903. (For curriculum, see *Appendix 3*, p. 191.) The three-year Ph.G. curriculum replaced the two-year curriculum; and in 1927 it became the minimum education required by law to qualify for the Wisconsin licensing examination.

As resurrected in 1925, the three-year curriculum offered all that was included in the two-year program and strengthened it in several ways. A year of English became mandatory, a subject in which many students had been "deplorably deficient." Studies were increased in pharmacognosy, a field that had been on the rise as a pharmaceutical science. The laboratory component was strengthened by student access to 38 acres of pharmacobotanical gardens, which were part of the Pharmaceutical Experiment Station (f. 1913; see p. 144). Eight of the ten elective credits were to be earned outside of the departments of pharmacy, chemistry and botany—consistent with Kremers' conviction that a pharmacy student ought to attain a well-rounded education. As a further step toward aligning pharmaceutical education with standards of the University at large, the student's credit load was increased from 16 to 18 semester hours. (For details, see *Appendix 3*.) The WPhA Committee on the School of Pharmacy apparently found these changes unobjectionable, except to note that graduates still would be "woefully lacking in business training."[18] At Wisconsin as in pharmaceutical education nationally, the three-year curriculum mostly strengthened existing subjects, rather than expanding in new directions.

With adoption of a three-year minimum nationally, a standard baccalaureate degree for pharmacists became a more realistic goal. While Wisconsin had offered such a degree since 1892, it became *required* first at Ohio State (1925), then, within two years, also at the universities of Georgia, Nebraska, and Minnesota. The incipient trend generated studies and debate within the American Association of Colleges of Pharmacy, culminating in a decision to ask member-colleges to require a four-year curriculum of all matriculants no later than 1932. Gainsayers pointed to what they considered the modest educational demands of the average practice, in which backroom manufacture and quality testing of drugs were dwindling and polypharmacal prescription compounding was also losing ground.[19]

Proponents of the longer curriculum tended to focus instead on the desirability of a broader-based education for pharmacists as community leaders and as practitioners fully knowledgeable about the scientific advances represented by newer products such as biologicals, hormones and chemical specifics. Kremers supported this view but was thwarted. "If

Wisconsin stood alone in 1892," he reminded members of the state association, "she has been followed by practically all her sister state universities and, so far as a required four-year undergraduate course is concerned, has been left behind by several of these institutions."[20] However, he was not able to make his pioneering four-year curriculum a requirement until the University confronted the 1932 deadline set by the AACP for nationwide compliance.

The B.Sc. Program Becomes Mandatory

For a Wisconsin student, the curriculum for the newly required B.Sc. degree proved to be no sharp break with the past. Comparing the four-year curriculum (see *Appendix 3*, p. 193) with the three-year curriculum, the most striking changes appear to have been the addition of 10 credits of physics, a doubling of credits (from 2 to 4) of elementary prescription practice, a doubling of credits (from 3 to 6) in pharmaceutical botany, expansion of assaying from 1 credit to 4, and paring back pharmaceutical technology from 8 credits to 5. To assure a good reading knowledge of *both* French and German, up to 28 credits was allotted (instead of 24) unless proficiency could be demonstrated by examination. A single credit was added to the electives (11 credits). And a series of lectures devoted to orientation in pharmacy added one credit. An improved curricular structure can be seen in the four-year sequence. Then as now, ongoing improvements within individual courses often were significant, yet leave only obscure traces in the record.

Three years after national adoption of the new standard, Kremers retired as Director of the School, vindicated in his decades of advocacy of a baccalaureate program comparable to programs in related fields—and unrepentant for his traditional statement in University catalogs that, "The object of the Course in Pharmacy is to furnish a thoroughly scientific foundation for the pursuit of the profession of pharmacy in all its branches." But Kremers had long since discovered a reality of academia, which he learned the hard way: "The task of the curriculum maker is simple enough," he said, "if, as an individual, he sits down to put his ideas on paper. It ceases to be simple when he attempts to carry out his ideas in practice. It becomes more complex if he has to satisfy his colleagues. It becomes a practical impossibility if he attempts to please all members of the profession. . . ."[21]

Changes in a curriculum often are stimulated by the vision of a School's director. That was true of Kremers; and, not surprisingly, a year after Arthur H. Uhl succeeded him as Director (1935; see p. 173), some

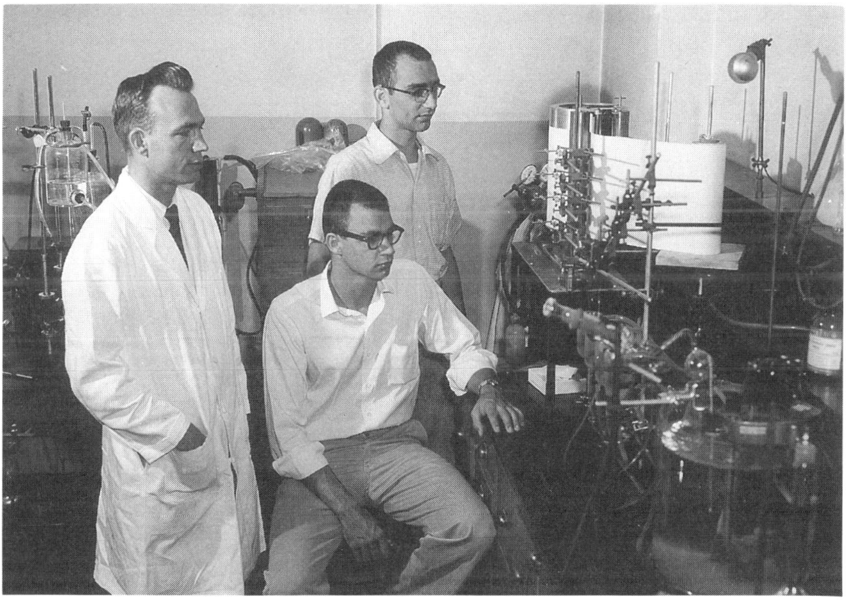

During the 1950s, traditional instruction in materia medica evolved into modern pharmacology, which became a major curricular area in the School by the 1970s. This laboratory scene, typical of the period, shows students watching a kymograph record drug effects on isolated uterine muscle. The supervising pharmacologist, Jack Miller (left), was on loan part-time from the medical faculty.

modifications of the four-year program were installed. For example, total semester-credits were increased from 120 to 128; botany credits were cut in half (to 5 credits), substituting zoology for the other 5 credits; prescription practice doubled (from 2 to 4 credits); pharmaceutical technology was cut back by a fifth (5 to 4 credits); electives were reduced (from 11 to 6 or 8 credits). Kremers' conviction about requiring both French and German (not shared by many undergraduates) now was relaxed to a total "language requirement" of 8 credits.[22]

Further curricular revision, six years later, added courses in bacteriology (4 credits), physiology (4 credits), and materia medica reappeared as a course (3 credits) separated from pharmacognosy and reinforced by some modern pharmacology.

Although pharmacy graduates now went forth armed with a science-based baccalaureate degree, their place in medical care was scarcely clarified. An after-effect of the industrial revolution was removing the preparation of dosage forms from community pharmacies, as it had earlier removed the preparation of the individual ingredients of dosage forms. Goaded by uncertainties, both professional and economic, organized pharmacy recruited the American Council on Education to undertake a remark-

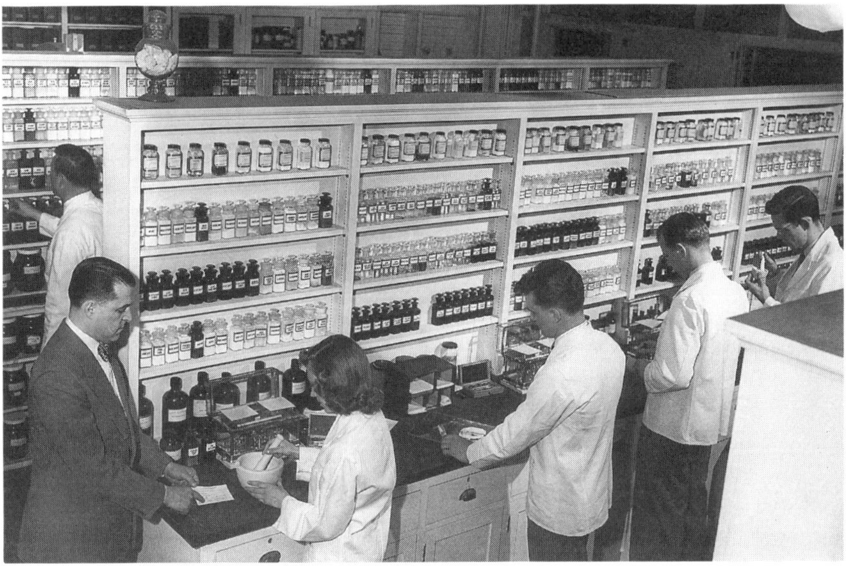

The laboratory setting for dispensing instruction during the 1940s (above) looked much as it had for several decades. A student is being helped with a prescription assignment by Professor Dale Wurster. Facilities were much improved in 1954 (below) when the dispensing laboratory was moved and modernized.

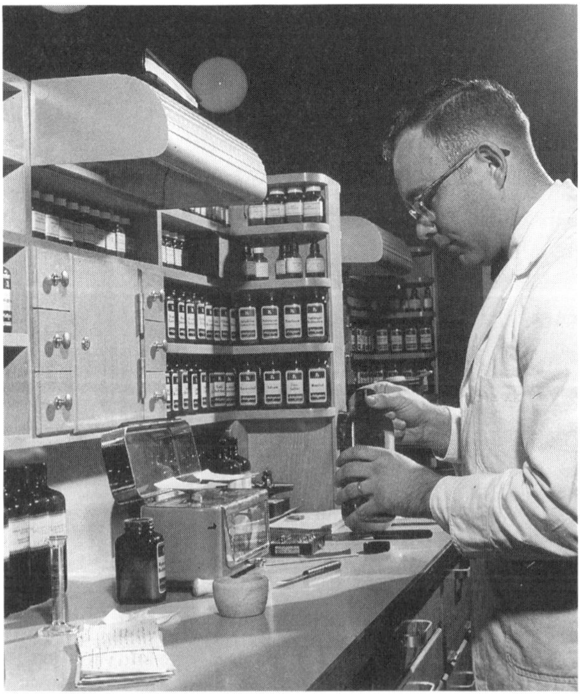

able national study of the profession and its educational system during the 1940s.[23] The resultant "Pharmaceutical Survey 1946–49" made a recommendation that influenced curricular development at Wisconsin and elsewhere. It held that educators should "continue their efforts for the constructive betterment of the existing four-year program of education," but also should "take the necessary initial steps for the development and establishment of a six-year program of education and training leading to the professional degree of Doctor of Pharmacy (Pharm.D.), this program to include two or more years of general education and basic science training."[24]

This ambivalent conclusion reflected divided opinion about curriculum length, both among the deans of the schools and in American pharmacy at large;[25] and it fostered, inadvertently, a movement nationally toward a five-year curriculum as a compromise. A five-year program, including two pre-professional years, had been advocated as early as 1930 by Frederick J. Wulling, Dean at the University of Minnesota,[26] which he thought "will not be difficult" to establish, but the idea was stillborn in a time when some schools of pharmacy had not even implemented a four-year baccalaureate.

A Five-Year Curriculum as Compromise

By the 1940s a five-year program no longer seemed radical, but remained controversial because for some it seemed too long for a baccalaureate degree, if indeed needed at all; for others it seemed too short to give pharmacy a fully professional basis and too short to justify a professional doctorate. The national Pharmaceutical Survey itself concluded that, "While a five-year program would overcome some of the limitations of the present [four-year] arrangement, it would leave much to be desired."[27] At Wisconsin, the Director said he was "never very happy about" the prospect of a five-year curriculum.[28] But several other schools adopted an optional curriculum of five years (including one or two preprofessional years). Ohio State University was the first to make five years of study mandatory, beginning with admissions in the fall of 1948. By 1952 thirteen other schools had adopted a five-year B.Sc. program, either optional or required;[29] Wisconsin stood among the schools for which it remained an unacceptable compromise.

Two years later the American Association of Colleges of Pharmacy voted to recommend a five-year baccalaureate as the minimum standard for students graduating after April 1, 1965.[30] Thus forewarned, the Wisconsin pharmacy faculty voted (1956) to move toward an extended curriculum.[31] Prospective students were informed that, to conform to the regulation of the American Council on Pharmaceutical Education, "a student who begins college training in or after April, 1960, as a candidate for the Bachelor of Science degree in Pharmacy, enters the School of Pharmacy at the beginning of the junior year after completing two years of work in the College of Letters and Science . . ." —to embark upon three years of professional studies.[32] Thus ended the four-year baccalaureate that Kremers had pioneered 68 years before as an optional curriculum.

Wisconsin students who enrolled in the new five-year curriculum (158 credits) encountered not only additional courses, but a restructured content in various courses from the old curriculum. *In the two prepharmacy years*, electives increased from 0 to 15 credits (about half of the additional year in the curriculum); chemistry increased from 10 to 18 credits; foreign language was removed as an alternative to the study of mathematics; physics was up from 0 to 6 credits; economics up from 0 to 3 credits; and botany substituted for half the zoology credits. This added up to a second year of pre-pharmacy study. The concept of pre-pharmacy study had been invoked (as the first of four years) when the School of Pharmacy became

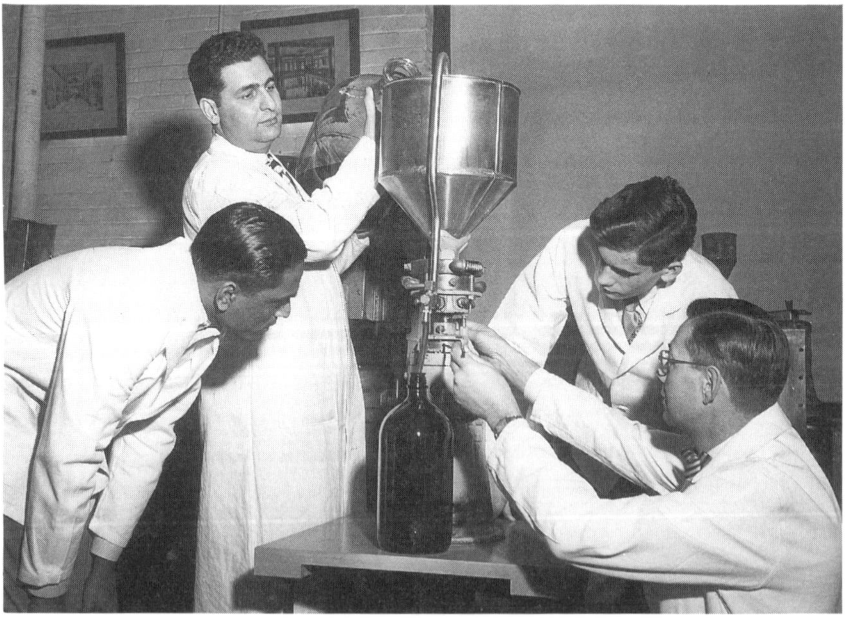

Pharmaceutical manufacturing was part of an elective industrial sequence in the early 1950s. Here Professor Louis Busse (right) is demonstrating a filtration process, assisted by William S. Apple (who later became Executive Director of the American Pharmaceutical Association).

independent of the College of Letters and Science in 1950. Even before that date the first year of the four-year program was devoted to general education and basic science courses; but it was not designated pre-professional because the College of Letters and Science viewed the entire four-year program as just one of many B.Sc. programs offered under its jurisdiction.

In the three professional years: materia medica became pharmacology, with credits increased from 4 to 7; pharmacognosy was up from 6 to 10 credits; pharmaceutical chemistry down from 29 to 18 credits; pharmacy administration up from 0 to 2 credits; and pharmacy/pharmaceutics down from 27 to 24 credits. However, a student also could draw upon the latter two subjects for 10 or 11 of the 16 course credits needed to construct the required "Technical Electives" unit. The constellation of courses for such a unit had to be selected according to the career "track" chosen: community pharmacy, hospital pharmacy, or industrial pharmacy. For details of the courses required in this initial five-year program, see *Appendix 3*, p. 195.

Since the 1940s, Wisconsin's pharmaceutics group, motivated by Takeru Higuchi, had pioneered applications of physical chemistry to pharmaceutical systems (as the University of California did also). By the 1950s "physical pharmacy" concepts were having a marked and lasting impact on undergraduate instruction at Wisconsin and, eventually, at many other schools.[33] Wisconsin's role in bringing a significant new dimension (i.e., "physical pharmacy") to the preparation of drugs probably delayed faculty recognition of the impact that the bio-sciences could have on pharmaceutical education. However, it was a harbinger of change in 1950–51 when for the first time a pharmacologist (recruited part-time from the Medical School) taught the Materia Medica course. The course description itself implied a transition to modern pharmacology, which was made explicit in the new five-year curriculum and was underscored by appointment in 1962 of Dr. Kenneth Finger as the first full-time pharmacologist on the pharmacy faculty.

In 1971 the faculty upgraded the curriculum when its Curriculum Committee advocated "more biological and disease-state emphasis" and "patient involvement." The far-reaching changes reorganized pharmaceutics as a five-semester sequence, giving less emphasis to traditional compounding techniques; expanded and restructured pharmacology into a three-semester sequence, leading into new courses on therapeutics, on therapeutic drug interactions, and on pharmaceutical toxicology; and also added a clinical clerkship (6 credits); pharmaceutical biochemistry (4 cred-

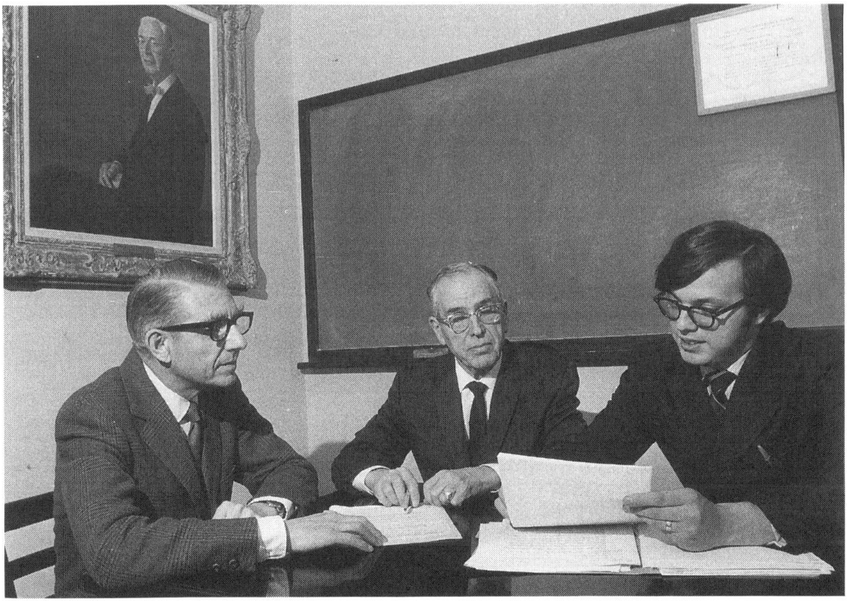

As a national center for cultivating and preserving pharmacy's history, the University has offered historical courses since 1906. A later generation of historians of pharmacy, Glenn Sonnedecker and John Parascandola, here discuss a project in 1970 with Dean Arthur Uhl (center).

its); pharmacy management (3 credits); social aspects of pharmacy (2 credits) and calculus.

Eighteen elective credits replaced the three professional "tracks" featured in the initial five-year program, to permit more individualized programs, a flexibility for which many students had petitioned. With the disappearance of the required unit of "Technical Electives," the revised curriculum altered considerably the amount of course work drawn from each of the five "curricular areas": Pharmaceutics was reduced from 23 to 16 credits; pharmaceutical chemistry and pharmacognosy together decreased from 26 to 18; while clinical pharmacy was up from 0 to 19; biological sciences increased from 18 to 26; pharmacy administration, including historical and social studies, went from 5 to 11.[34] The two credits of "social pharmacy" added to the curriculum marked the modest beginning of a new way of looking at contemporary pharmacy in American teaching, on which graduate research had been initiated already in 1963. It was a sociologic counterpart of the instruction and research in "historical pharmacy," which Wisconsin had pioneered since the turn of the century. As social studies of pharmacy matured and gained its own chair in the faculty (1975), the concept generated a curricular influence nationally.[35]

Impact of Clinical Pharmacy

The three-year professional sequence continued to evolve under the influence of internal evaluations of instruction, changing accreditation standards, and national studies sponsored during the 1970s by the AACP and APhA.[36] A common theme that emerged and had a pervasive impact on undergraduate instruction was "clinical pharmacy" as a national aspiration and mode of practice. Its modest local debut in 1966–67 had been an "initial trial of an experimental course with four students."[37] The faculty's view of the curriculum gradually shifted toward a clinical orientation, but it was hard to implement fully without having the extra year afforded at schools that adopted a six-year program.

As early as 1948 the Pharmacy Division of the Wisconsin faculty had developed on paper an optional six-year curriculum; and Dean Uhl told the Vice President of Academic Affairs the following year that, "In accordance with the recommendation of the Pharmaceutical Survey and the American Association of Colleges of Pharmacy, steps will be taken for the

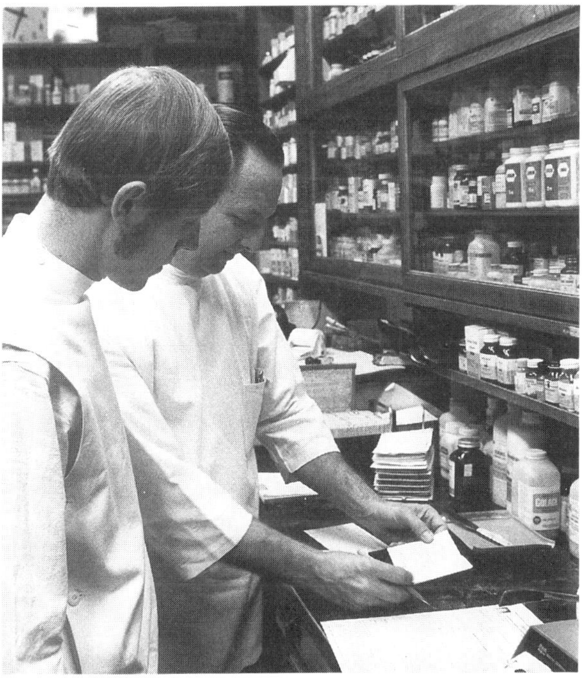

The externship was where the curriculum connected with the "real world" for this pharmacy student of the 1970s. The pharmacist-preceptor (at right) was Jack Werts in Madison.

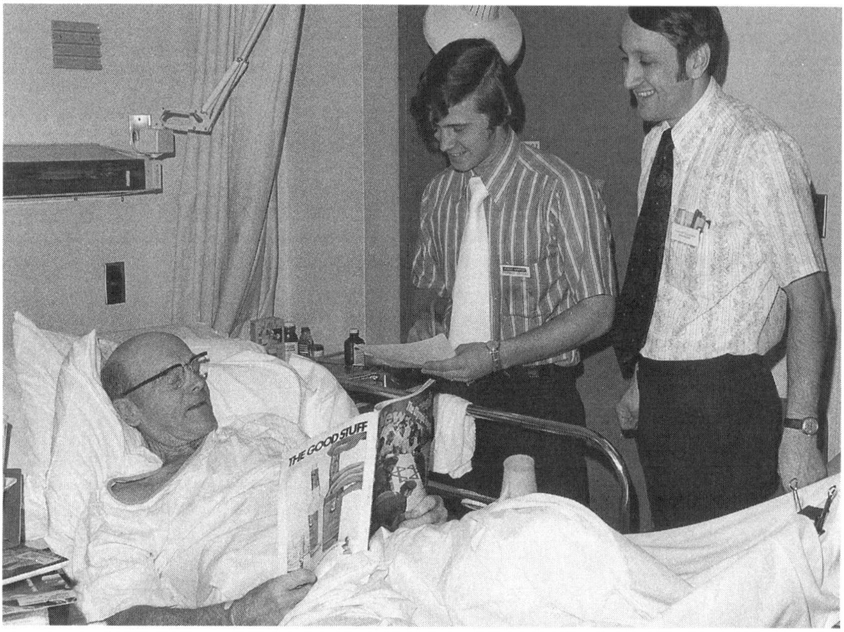

Clinical pharmacy had become an important part of the curriculum for these students, shown on the wards of University Hospital in the early 1970s.

development and establishment of a six-year program . . . on a voluntary basis as soon as it is possible to do so."[38] That time never came for Dean Uhl. A quarter century later, however, the concept of a curriculum leading to the Doctor of Pharmacy degree was given new impetus by a Committee on the Future of the School. Unlike the aborted curricular plan of 1948, the new proposal was shaped by a clinical focus, and it received a unanimous vote of support from the pharmacy faculty in 1974.[39] This was a curriculum designed for the few rather than the many (i.e., five to ten students), for a student who wanted to become a "differentiated" specialist rather than a generalist. A "Doctor of Pharmacy" candidate would be expected to have a B.Sc. degree as the prerequisite to two or three years of advanced professional studies, a "strong residency" and the possibility of specialization (permitting discontinuance of the existing M.Sc. program in hospital pharmacy). The program would be administered by the School of Pharmacy, not the Graduate School (an earlier bone of contention). When the University again delayed implementation, the School again resorted to strengthening the clinical component of the existing five-year B. Sc., and inaugurated "block" scheduling by the half semester, to permit a more effective clinical clerkship (1977–78; see *Appendix 3*, p. 196).[40] It was not enough. The American Council on Pharmaceutical Education issued a negative report on the adequacy of Wisconsin's clinical program, following an on-site inspection (1980). The School's Task Force on Clinical Education and Training prepared proposals that were expected to satisfy the ACPE concerns.[41]

It was still not enough. In 1982 the ACPE placed Wisconsin's accreditation in probationary status, although that was never announced publicly because of remedial measures promptly initiated. For a school often told that it was one of the leaders, this episode was painful; but by the end of the School's centenary year the accreditation cloud had lifted.[42]

Epilogue to the First Century

The final year of the B.Sc. curriculum underwent "profound changes," culminating with innovations in the fall of 1982, as the School's first century drew toward its close.[43] But Dean August Lemberger reminded the faculty that it was no long-range solution to the curricular issue and that the UW was "the only Big 10 school of pharmacy that did not have an approved Doctor of Pharmacy program." Thus challenged, the faculty approved in 1984 several major initiatives put forward by a Task Force on Advanced Professional Education. The Task Force then developed *three* curricula, for which the University eventually authorized three new degree designations:

1 A seven-year optional program leading to a Doctor of Pharmacy degree. In the fall of 1990 the first six students enrolled. Students were required to have four years of pre-Pharm.D. studies (128 credits) preparatory to the three-year professional sequence (90 credits). Objective: To qualify selected students for the highest levels of practice, including specialized roles in clinical pharmacy.

2 A four-year optional program leading to a B.Sc. in Pharmacology and Toxicology. In the fall of 1985 the first six students enrolled. Objective: To prepare selected students to advance into a Ph.D. program or into laboratory jobs requiring their special skills.

3 A four-year optional program leading to a B.Sc. in Pharmaceutical Sciences. In the fall of 1990 the first 14 students enrolled. Objective: To qualify a student to advance into a doctoral program, whether professional (Pharm.D.) or research (Ph.D.), into some other professional school, or into the marketplace for a technical laboratory position.

Of the three new curricula, only the "Pharm.D.' qualified a student to take the state examination for a license to practice pharmacy. For that purpose, most students would continue to enroll in the five-year B.Sc. program. Although the Pharm.D. curriculum was approved by the pharmacy faculty in December 1985, it would be another five years before the last bureaucratic hurdle was surmounted and the first students were at work.[44] In the enthusiasm of a long-delayed success, perhaps no one foresaw that Wisconsin's Pharm.D. curriculum set a standard too high to be sustained. As the School moved deeper into its second century, beyond range of the present account, plans called for converting to a six-year curriculum[45] (206 credits in 2 + 4 years), designed for a higher level of "pharmaceutical care." Yet, as in a century past, the new curriculum will someday be superseded, as the uncertainties of another century unfold.

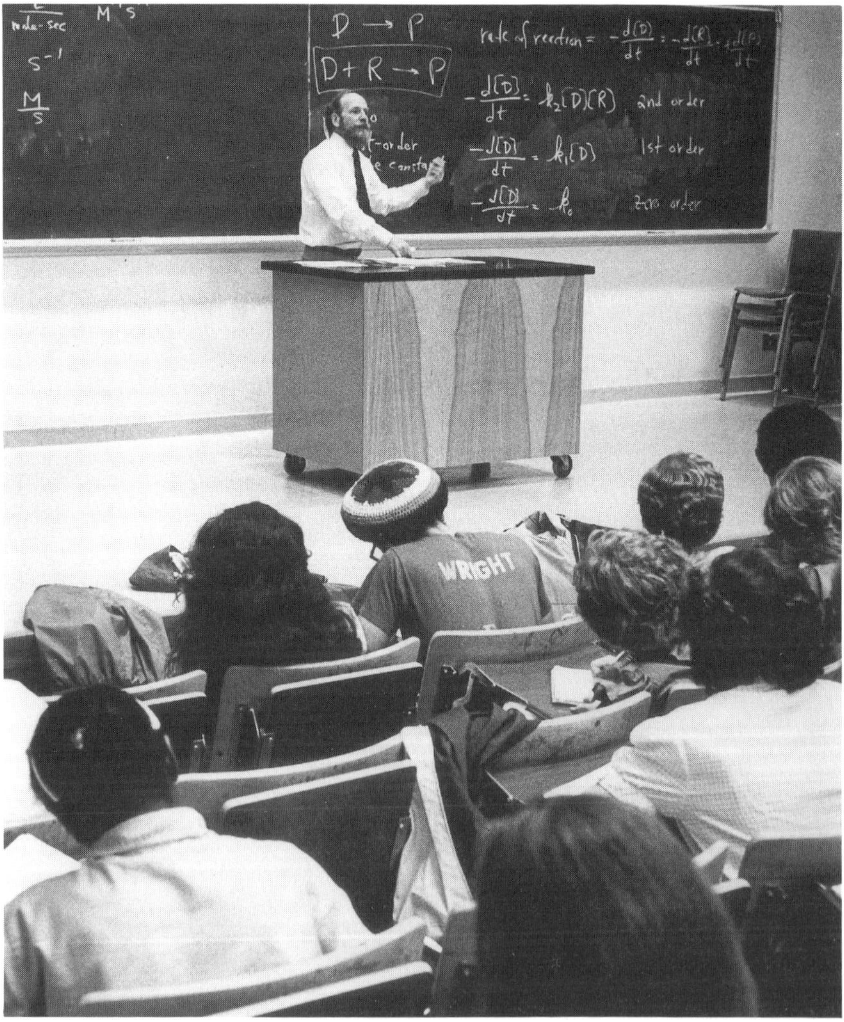

The complexities of pharmaceutical analysis hold the attention of students during a lecture by Professor Kenneth Connors about 1980.

Notes and References

1. Folios 42–48 of the manuscript preserved at the Wellcome Institute for the History of Medicine, London. Power apparently took the notebook with him when he left Wisconsin (1892) to enter industry and, later, when he left for England to become Director of the Wellcome Chemical Research Laboratories. Long forgotten among Power's personal papers, the notebook was identified by Prof. John K. Crellin while at the Wellcome Institute (now at St. John's University in Newfoundland), who kindly called it to our attention and arranged for the purchase of a photocopy, through the courtesy of the Library of the Wellcome Institute for the History of Medicine. The notebook is identified on the flyleaf, "Fred. B. Power, Phila. College of Pharmacy, 145 W. 10th St."
2. Recollection of Edward Kremers, in "Dr. Power at Wisconsin," *Badger Pharmacist*, 1936, No. 13, 5.
3. *Announcement*, . . .1883–84, 6. It also lists the textbooks utilized. For examples of some of the better Senior theses or essays, see *Contributions from the Department of Pharmacy*, No. 1, 1885, 61 pp., and No. 2, 1986, 52 pp.
4. Edward Kremers, "Pharmaceutical Education by the State," *Wis. Drugg.*, Oct. 1935, 3.
5. Edward Kremers, "President's Address," *ACPF, Proc. 1903–04*, 4.
6. George Urdang, "Edward Kremers, Reformer of American Pharmaceutical Education," *Am. J. Pharm. Educ.* 11 (1947): 631–658. *Catalogue for 1893–1894*, 182.
7. Recounted to me about 1950 by Professor George Urdang, who had been a close associate of Kremers. It is a remark characteristic of Kremers, even if the incident cannot be confirmed.
8. *Catalogue . . .1893–1894*, 182.
9. *Proc. WPhA, 1893*, 17–19. Speaking in August 1893, Kremers alluded to the "four years' course offered since last year [i.e., 1892], and explained that ". . .Since the course could not be advertised in the last year's Announcement [of courses], no students were anticipated. However two students entered the same last fall. . . ." (Ibid., 20).
10. Ibid., 34 f. At this time, up to fourteen months of the apprenticeship requirement could be absolved by an equivalent amount of pharmaceutical study at the UW. For a review of Association involvement, see Edwin J. Boberg, "Summary of School of Pharmacy Committees' Reports," *Proc. WPhA, 1930*, 83.
11. Wisconsin Laws of 1882, Ch., 167, Sec. 4. Eunice Bonow Bardell, *Wisconsin Show Globe* (Madison, 1983), 24.
12. *Fifteenth Annual Report of the Wisconsin Board of Pharmacy, 1896*, 3. Until the pharmacy law revision of 1927, the Assistant Pharmacists registered annually far outnumbered the Pharmacists registered. ("State Board of Pharmacy," *Badger Pharmacist*, No. 17 (Aug.) 1937, 21. A.L.I. Winne, "Abolishing the Assistant Grade," *J. Am. Pharm. Assoc.* 19 (1930): 397 f.
13. "Report of the School of Pharmacy," *Proc. WPhA 1901*, 52–54. By 1903 Milwaukee was offering curricula of two, three and four years in length. But the advent of World War I reduced the number of pharmacy students to six. Soon thereafter the Department closed, never to reopen. (Sol R. Bear, "The History of the School of Pharmacy at the Marquette University School of Pharmacy," B.Sc. (Pharm.) thesis, University of Wisconsin, 1950. 18 pp.)

14. State of New York, Education Department, *Handbook 11: Higher Education. Pharmacy. . .* , n.p., July 1907, 7; referring to Laws of New York, Ch. 667, Sec. 194(6). National use of *The Pharmaceutical Syllabus* was aborted in 1946 out of fear that it was becoming obligatory as a curricular standard.
15. *Proc. WPhA 1923*, 51 f. Earlier, Kremers had nettled WPhA members by asking rhetorically, "What might have been the progress if in place of indifference and hostility we had enjoyed your sympathy and support?" Ibid., 1911, 40.
16. In 1926 pharmacist Oscar Rennebohm of Madison goaded his fellow WPhA members with a stark fact, that "Wisconsin is the only state in the Old Northwest that has not a college prerequisite" for licensure. ("Report on the School of Pharmacy," *Proc. WPhA 1926*, 110, also 79). A year later a revised pharmacy law made graduation from a three-year curriculum prerequisite to taking Wisconsin's licensing examination. (Bardell, (n. 11), 95–99). The Conference (ACPF), which became the American Association of Colleges of Pharmacy (AACP) in 1925, tried to foster modest minimum standards prior to the founding of a separate accreditation agency in 1932, the American Council on Pharmaceutical Education (ACPE).
17. *Catalog . . . 1925–26*, 94.
18. *Course in Pharmacy 1927–28, Bulletin*, April 1927, 10 and 12. "Personal Report of the Chairman . . .," *Proc. WPhA 1924*, 168.
19. According to one estimate, "on the average [pharmacists] compound only about 1,200 prescriptions per year . . ." (*Medical Care for the American People; the Final Report of the Committee on the Costs of Medical Care* (Chicago: University of Chicago, 1932), 28 f.)
20. "Address by President Edward Kremers," *Proc. WPhA 1930*, 28.
21. "Address by Dr. Edward Kremers," *Proc. WPhA 1929*, 120.
22. *Catalogue, 1936–37*, 80.
23. A section on "The Pharmaceutical Curriculum" (pp.98–107) was included in The *General Report of the Pharmaceutical Survey*, Edward C. Elliott, Director (Washington: American Council on Education, c. 1950), 240 pp. A separate monograph devoted entirely to curriculum became too controversial for publication under the Survey imprimatur. See Robert G. Mrtek, "Pharmaceutical Education in These United States—An Interpretive Historical Essay of the Twentieth Century," *Am. J. Pharmaceu. Edu.* 40 (1976): 355 f.
24. *General Report*, (n. 23), 229 f.
25. Ibid., 104 f. The Director of the Survey noted that "At no other point has there been sharper differences of judgment among the profession. The issues involve what should be taught, how much, when, and to whom." (ibid., 98) One notable deficiency reported was "woefully inadequate instruction in pharmacology and pharmacy administration."
26. Frederick J. Wulling, "Completion of the Junior College the Next Prerequisite," *J. Am. Pharm. Assoc.* 19 (1930): 394–397; also 20 (1931): 786–789. Minnesota had 18 students enrolled at the time in an optional five-year program.
27. *General Report*, (n. 23), 105.
28. Arthur H. Uhl, Oral History Project interview, June 1974, ms, 24, Archives.
29. Joseph B. Burt, Chair, "Report of the Executive Committee, AACP, 1951–52," *Am. J. Pharmaceu. Edu.* 16 (1952): 574.

30. Mrtek, "Pharmaceutical Education," (n. 23), 356, summarizes the AACP maneuvers leading up to this decision. See also Lloyd E. Blauch and George L. Webster, *The Pharmaceutical Curriculum* (Washington, c. 1952), 28–44. Both the APhA and NABP concurred, and the recommendation was adopted as part of the accreditation standards by the American Council on Pharmaceutical Education.

31. Minutes, School of Pharmacy Faculty, meeting January 16, 1956, Kremers Reference Files (KRF), "C31(a)I:Wis., 1950s." Such a major change became less complicated to achieve after the School of Pharmacy separated from the College of Letters and Science, in 1950, as a professional school with its own Dean.

32. *Announcement, 1958–60*, 13. Considerable insight concerning conditions in, and hopes for, the undergraduate program during the 1960s can be gained from the document, "Committee on Internal Study of Teaching and of Faculty-Student Relationships in the School of Pharmacy—Report of a Special Committee" (G. Sonnedecker, Chair) June 1967, 82 pp. (in KRF at "C31(a)I:Wisconsin").

33. Blauch and Webster, (n. 30), 145–147; and Joseph V. Swintosky, "A Half Century in Pharmaceutical Science and Education," *Am. J. Pharmaceu. Edu.* 54 (1990): 383–389. *Announcement . . . 1950–52*, 460.

34. The revision of the curriculum was approved by the Pharmacy Faculty March 22, 1971, and by other UW bodies that spring, as required. Dean Perlman projected stepwise implementation during the ensuing two years or so. D. Perlman to Pharmacy Faculty, "Implementation . . .," 3-p. memo; and "Final Curriculum Proposal," Curriculum Committee to the Pharmacy Faculty, March 11, 1971—both in KRF, "C31(a):Wis., 1970s." The latter features syllabi for individual courses as revised by the respective instructors.

35. On the early years, see "Social Studies of Pharmacy—An Invitational Conference Sponsored by the University of Wisconsin, November 1969," *Amer. J. Pharmaceu. Edu.*, 34 (1970): 529–586. First occupant of the first full-time chair for a pharmaceutical sociologist in the USA was Bonnie L. Svarstad; first occupant of the first full-time chair for a historian of pharmacy (1947) was George Urdang, brought to Wisconsin earlier by Edward Kremers as his collaborator, initially as co-author of a book, *History of Pharmacy; a Guide and a Survey*.

36. Among studies particularly influential were: (1) "Committee on Internal Study of Teaching and of Faculty-Student Relationships in the [UW] School of Pharmacy—Report of a Special Committee," June 1967, 82 pp.; (2) *Pharmacists for the Future—The Report of the Study Commission on Pharmacy* (Ann Arbor: Health Administration Press, c. 1975), 161 pp.; (3) M. Rosenfeld, et al., eds., *A National Study of the Practice of Pharmacy* (Washington: APhA, 1978), 108 pp.; (4) "Curricular Affairs Subcommittee Report, Self-Study Committee," [UW] School of Pharmacy, 1979) and the School's "Self-Study Report. . . to the American Council on Pharmaceutical Education," March 1980 (in KRF, "C31(a)I:Wis. 1980").

37. David Perlman, Coordinator, in a grant proposal to the National Institutes of Health, 1969, 33, KRF, "C31(a)I:Wis., 1960s." On the beginnings nationally see "Clinical Pharmacy in Historical Perspective," *Drug Intell. & Clin. Pharm.* 10 (1976): 505–527.

38. A.H. Uhl to Ira L. Baldwin, June 4, 1949; Pharmacy Division to the Curriculum Committee, "The Pharmacy Courses of the Six-Year Curriculum," n.d., 3 pp.; Louis W. Busse to the Division, 2 pp.; "Preliminary Report of the Curriculum Committee on a Proposed Six-Year Program," December 29, 1948, 3 pp.—all in KRF, "C31(a)I:Wis., 1940s."
39. "Progress Report. . .Committee on the Future of the School," Kenneth A. Connors, Chair, March 6, 1974, 2 pp. The Committee's "Report on a Doctor of Pharmacy Program" is Faculty Document No. 020175, July 5, 1974, 2 pp.—both in KRF, "C31(a)I:Wis., 1970s."
40. Minutes, Pharmacy Faculty, March 31, 1977, and Pharmacy Alumni Association Newsletter, Winter 1982, 3 f.
41. ACPE, "Report on the Program Leading to the Degree of Bachelor of Science in Pharmacy . . .," March 11–13, 1980, 15 f.; "Final Report of the Task Force on Clinical Education and Training," June 2, 1980, School of Pharmacy; "Minutes," Pharmacy Faculty, December 18, 1980—all in KRF, "C31(a)I:Wis.,1980s."
42. ACPE, "Action and Recommendations of the American Council on Pharmaceutical Education for the Baccalaureate Program in Pharmacy at the University of Wisconsin School of Pharmacy, January 14–16, 1983," in KRF, "C31(a)I:Wis., 1980s." Unpublicized probation was one of the measures that ACPE had available (at that time) to help rectify curable deficiencies in a school's compliance with national standards. For additional details about the tortuous route taken by the School toward a Doctor of Pharmacy program, see research notes compiled by Gregory J. Higby as appreciated assistance to the present project: "Clinical Pharmacy c. 1967–83," c. 1983, 8 pp. in KRF, "C31(a)I:Wis.,1970s."
43. The *Bulletin . . . School of Pharmacy*, (No. 7, September 1982, 8) announced the details of the further revision of the five-year (B.Sc.) program, beginning with the academic year 1982–83. Changes were introduced in the sequencing and credits of old courses, and new courses were offered on dosage forms, physical pharmacy, drug-delivery systems, and clinical pharmacokinetics.
44. At this time, 39 of the 72 USA schools had a Pharm. D. program in operation or in process of accreditation. A. P. Lemberger, "School of Pharmacy Report," *Wisconsin Pharmacist*, Nov. 1984, 349, and *Pharmacy Alumni Newsletter*, No. 95, 1985, 1; "[Revised] Report: Task Force on Advance Professional Education," Christine Sorkness, Chair, 16 Dec. 1985, KRF. "C31(a)I:1980s"; and Chris Sorkness, "The Future of the Doctor of Pharmacy Program at the University of Wisconsin," *Mortar & Quill* (UW School of Pharmacy) 23 (1987): 2–4. To illustrate the cumbersome process of change: After the University administration "granted a preliminary entitlement to plan . . . on September 30, 1986, the proposals for the two new curricula [four-year B.Sc. Pharm. Sci. and seven-year Pharm.D.] were approved by the University Academic Planning Council . . . In March 1987, these curricula were also approved by the Madison campus Faculty Senate." Subsequently, the proposals were reviewed by the University of Wisconsin System, then approved by the University Board of Regents. (Minutes, Pharmacy Faculty, Dec. 16, 1988).
45. "Summary . . . Faculty Retreat," Devil's Head, Wis., Aug. 24–25, 1995, and *Pharmacy Graduate* (Pharmacy Alumni Association), Fall 1995, 1. At this time, twenty-eight of the seventy-five USA accredited schools were offering the Pharm.D. as the only professional degree. *AACP Newsletter*, Jan. 1996, 13.

CHAPTER 4

The Students

BY CARL BUCKNER

PHARMACY STUDENTS have brought to the University diverse backgrounds. Here they found a campus-wide, heterogeneous community of fellow students[1] in which to interact, grow, and change their thought, and ideas. How this inner life of students has affected the post-graduation outcome, in helping to create pharmacists and educated citizens, is historically significant but elusive. So, instead—given the spotty source material that survives and the limited space available—this chapter presents an overview of student activities and organizations in the School and relates them, where possible, to campus-wide events.

Enrollment

When the School of Pharmacy opened in 1883, 27 students enrolled.[2] Although this number of students seems small, pharmacy actually represented 7% of the total University population in that first year. In the following year, pharmacy enrollment reached 10.6% of that of the University, but declined relatively thereafter. By 1901–02, pharmacy students constituted only about 1% of the University enrollment, although the total pharmacy enrollment had stayed relatively constant since the beginning. In fact, the total enrollment remained at about the same level until the end of World War I (Figures 1 and 2).

The decline in percentage of pharmacy students around the turn of the century can be attributed largely to a more than seven-fold rise in the University population between 1883 and 1901. This was a period of dramatic growth in population and industry in the country. Recognition by some that a college education might be a prerequisite for success in the twentieth century helped boost enrollments across the nation. However,

FIGURE 1 - FIRST CENTURY ENROLLMENT IN PHARMACY COMPARED WITH CAMPUS-WIDE POPULATION

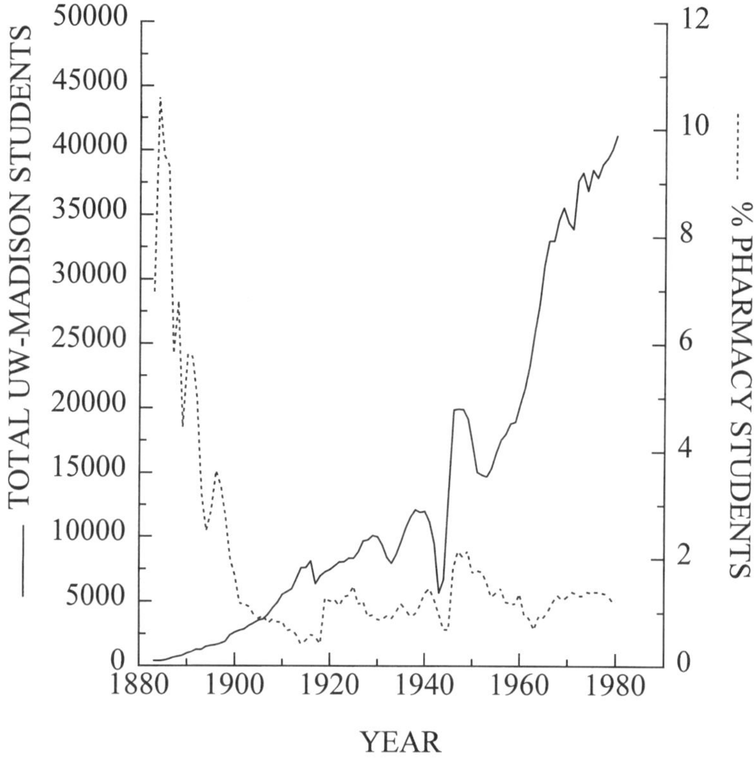

pharmacy enrollment at Wisconsin did not keep pace with the expansion of the University in the latter part of the nineteenth century. One brake on enrollment was recognition that a university degree was not necessary for pharmacy licensure and practice. Kremers himself tended to emphasize as factors the Spanish-American War and the stamp tax,[3] although these events did not appear to influence enrollment in the university as a whole or in at least one neighboring pharmacy school.[4] Enrollment in pharmacy remained around 30 to 50 students after the Spanish War when University enrollment continued to rise (Figure 2).

The first major jump in pharmacy enrollment came in the fall of 1919, when the number of students tripled from the previous year (Figure 2). This sharp growth can be largely attributed to an influx of World War I veterans. Although there was no automatic government scholarship avail-

FIGURE 2 - FIRST CENTURY ENROLLMENT OF FEMALES IN PHARMACY

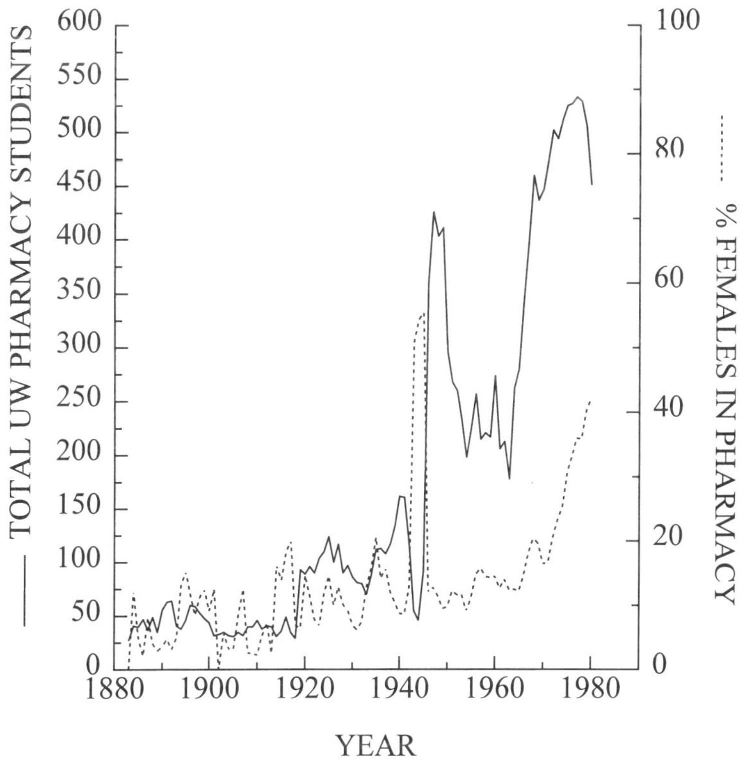

able to veterans, there was increased interest in education resulting from technological advances during the war. A close relationship between chemistry and medicine was beginning to be appreciated, and pharmacy was one of the beneficiaries. The percentage of pharmacy students at UW increased from 0.4% in 1918–19 to 1.3% in 1919–20.[5]

Although there was a small decline in the University population, pharmacy enrollment was not markedly altered during World War I (Figure 1). The U. S. Army, fearing a shortage of trainees in the health sciences and engineering as a result of the military draft, created the Students Army Training Corps (SATC) in 1918. Under this program, students drafted into the military could enroll in SATC and remain in school until they were needed for military duty. Many pharmacy students participated and this helped maintain enrollment in pharmacy.[6]

Pharmacy enrollment remained rather constant during the 1920s, but fell slightly along with the total University population (Figures 1 and 2) in the early 1930s due to the economic depression. After some sense of recovery was felt with the election of F. D. Roosevelt, enrollments at both levels took an upward trend beginning in 1934–35. However, these were still difficult economic times for students, and many worked overtime at menial jobs to earn their way.[7]

World War II drastically affected student populations everywhere. At Wisconsin, pharmacy student enrollment fell from a high of 162 in 1940–41 to a low of 46 in 1944–45 (Figures 1 and 2). Many students were drafted; others were eager to volunteer. Deferments for pharmacy students in the early years of the war helped prevent an initial sharp decline, but eventually a heavy impact was felt from the accelerated program of the School, the reluctance of many students to remain at home and the absence of deferments toward the end of the war.[8]

The sharpest rise in pharmacy enrollment in the history of the school occurred in 1946–47 when the flood of World War II veterans quadrupled the student population.[9] The percentage of pharmacy students at UW rose to 2.1% in 1947–48. These dramatic changes are readily apparent in

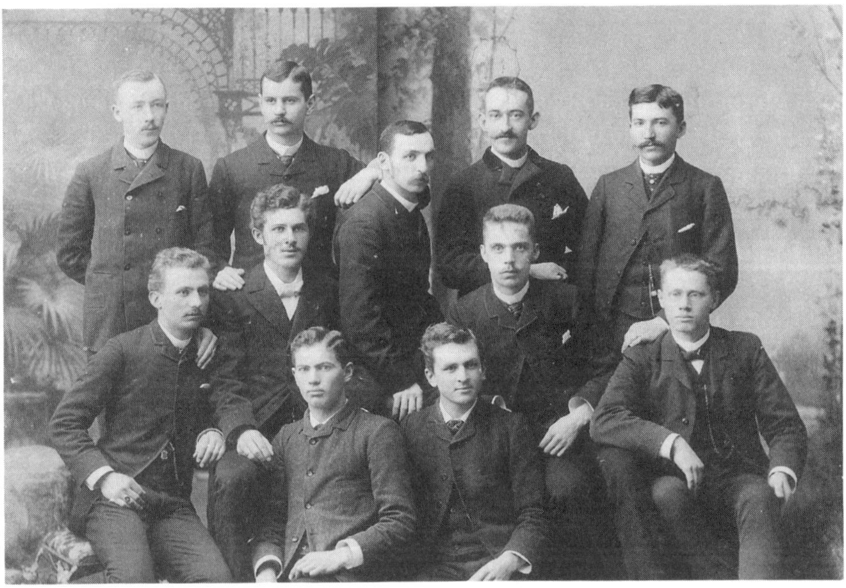

Pharmacy was a man's work (with few exceptions) when this Class of 1886 was photographed. The youth at the extreme lower right was to become one of the most distinguished American pharmacists of his time: Edward Kremers.

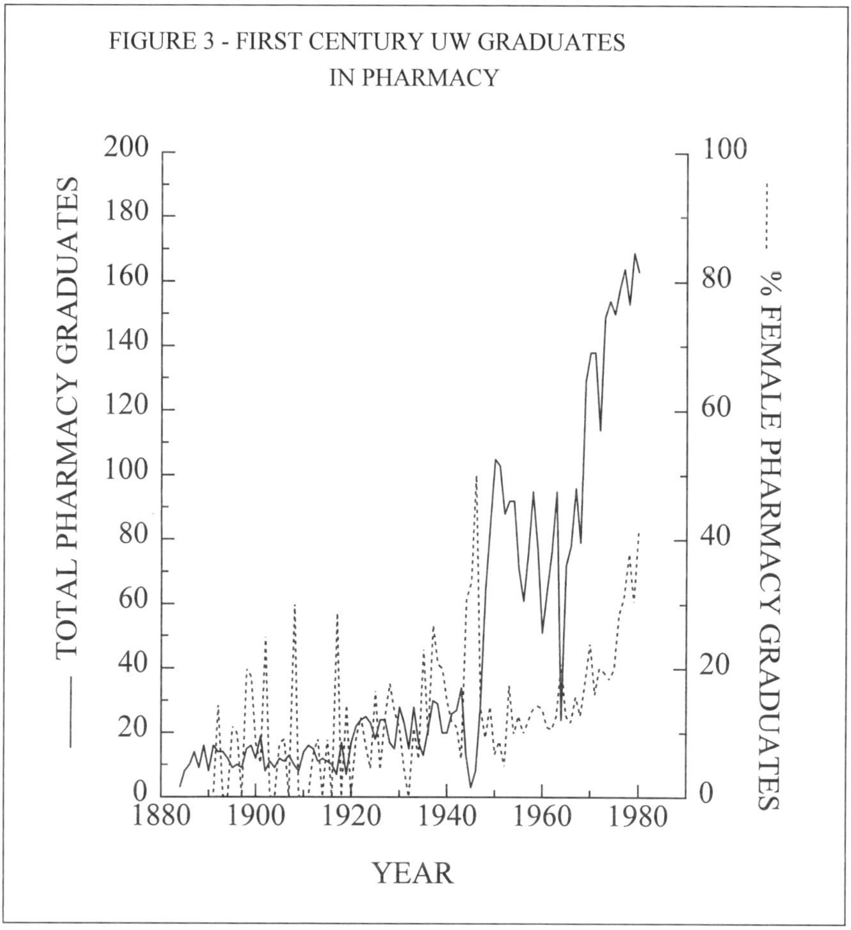

Figures 1, 2, and 3. Prompted by the "G.I. Bill of Rights" and the awesome growth in technology, especially in drug-related areas during the war, the veteran was eager to take advantage of the opportunities. The burgeoning student population created many shortages, especially in housing and classroom space, which continued throughout the decade.[10] This helped to make feasible, in 1947, the offering of the first year of the pharmacy course at the Milwaukee Extension Center.

The 1950s and early 1960s brought relative quiescence and stability, as the student population in pharmacy leveled off at about double that of the prewar period. The graduated veterans blended into suburbia, USA, to raise a coming generation of students.

The postwar "baby boom" contributed substantially to the upward turn of enrollment beginning in the mid–1960s. By 1970–71, the pharmacy student population had doubled that of the early 1960s, but remained around 1% of the total University population (Figure 1).

Pharmacy enrollment soared to an all-time high in 1977–78 (Figure 2). The increase during the 1970s can be attributed at least partially to "capitation" grants by the federal government in an attempt to increase the supply of health care practitioners (see Chapter 2, p. 60). Eventually, a perceived overabundance of pharmacists led to discontinuation of capitation grants and to declining enrollments in the late 1970s and early 1980s.

During most of its history, the School of Pharmacy (like most other departments in the University) has had a disproportionately small number of female and minority students. The plight of both groups was tied to social attitudes and conventions. For women, the question has been whether to attempt to succeed in a male-dominated business world at the expense of the stereotypical roles of wife and mother. For minorities, attempts to compete in a white-dominated society has been handicapped by the remnants of racism and economic disadvantages. By the 1990s both groups had made a major advance toward their rightful place in Wisconsin pharmacy.

After many years of sporadic debate, full coeducation on the Madison campus was finally supported by a resolution of the Board of Regents on January 21, 1874.[11] After that, resistance was meager. Nevertheless, the proportion of females among the students remained low. When the School of Pharmacy opened in 1883, the clientele was exclusively male. In subsequent years women began to enroll in pharmacy, but the first woman did not graduate from the school until 1892[12] (Figure 3).

The suffragist movement of the late nineteenth and early twentieth centuries did little to improve female enrollment in pharmacy. For example, in 1902–03 there were no women enrolled in the pharmacy curriculum (Figure 2). Graduation records show that, out of 850 graduates of the school up to 1940, only 76 (or 9%) were female. Before World War II, the percentage of women in the school of pharmacy fluctuated considerably, a peak of 21% being recorded in 1935–36. In many of those years, Wisconsin was slightly better than the national average among pharmacy schools. To some extent, this might be attributed to the presence on the faculty of Nellie Wakeman (see p. 140 and *Appendix 2*), who provided a "role model" and helped lead a national movement to increase the number of female pharmacists.[13] Also, as Director of the School, Kremers was not averse to the encouragement of women to enter the profession.[14] Nevertheless, in the male-dominated pharmacy world there seemed to be assumptions that women were inferior to men in capacity, and that the practice of pharmacy was not suitable work for women. It is understandable if some women were deterred.[15]

When World War II broke out, women across the nation began entering the work force in large numbers, and were viewed as fulfilling a national priority to maintain labor at home while allowing men to fight the war. For the first time, traditional life styles were widely shattered and many women found gratification in their new identities away from the home.[16]

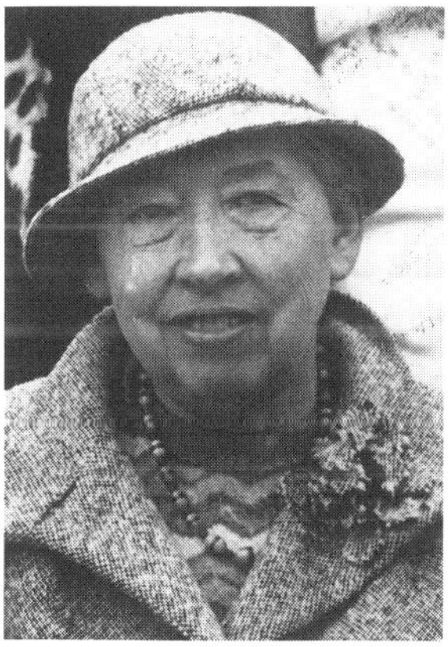

Female students were encouraged by friendly Prof. Nellie A. Wakeman, the first woman on the pharmacy faculty, 1913–46. She herself was the first female graduate to earn a Ph.D. at the School.

At Wisconsin, female pharmacy enrollment during the war was spurred by an attempt on the part of the school, with cooperation from the Wisconsin Pharmaceutical Association (WPhA), to interest a "minimum" number of women in attending.[17] The success of this program can be judged by the fact that the number of females enrolled in pharmacy doubled in the years 1943–44 and 1944–45, and doubled again in 1945–46. Even more dramatic, due to the wartime decline in the male population of the University, the percentage of females in pharmacy rose to slightly more than 50% in each of those years [18] (Figure 2).

The end of the war brought a decline in the percentage of females in the School, as the males returned from war. However, except for 1954–55, the actual number of women in the School stayed well above that of pre-war years.[19] Many of the old taboos had been erased and new modes of behavior were taking shape. Women liked the idea of working (at least part time) to supplement the family income in the face of inflation and increasing family desires; perhaps even more, they liked the new kind of freedom and identity outside the home. Their daughters were to cast aside traditional feminine roles still more readily, having witnessed the increasing degree of overlap of the domains of the two sexes.[20]

A dramatic rise in the number of female students at Wisconsin and across the nation began in the mid–1960s (Figure 2). This rise was not limited to pharmacy, but was part of a growing feminist movement, which saw equal opportunity as a basic human right.[21] Furthermore, the student movement of the late 1960s brought a new social consciousness, one which demanded equal treatment for all.[22]

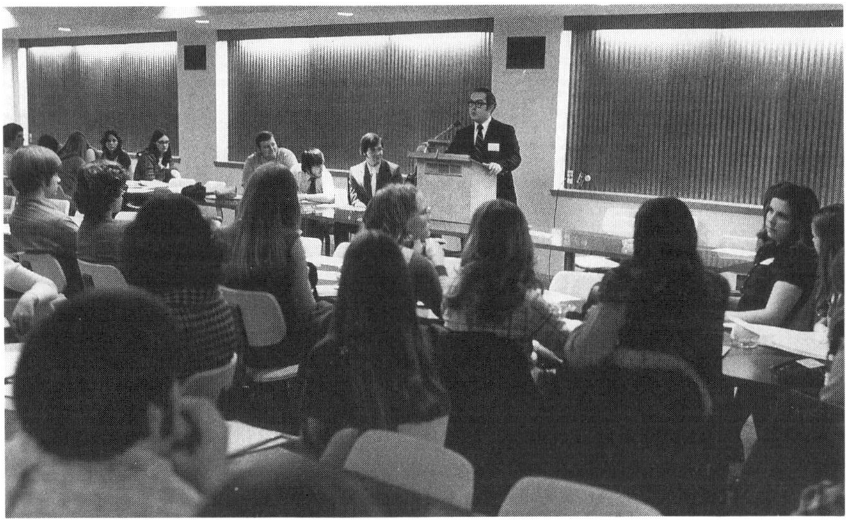

Annual recruitment efforts have maintained a high caliber of student enrollment in the School. No one expected the sparse female contingent among these visitors to the campus during the early 1970s to become within two decades a majority of the annual enrollment.

The student movement of the 1960s was probably a primary stimulus for development of programs to aid the acquisition and retention of minority students at Wisconsin. The actual number of minority students in the School of Pharmacy over the years of its existence is not available, but it certainly has never been large.[23] For example, in 1980 when the total minority enrollment in UW–Madison did not exceed 5%, minority enrollment in pharmacy reached 6.2%, largely due to the establishment of an effective minority affairs program with extramural funding.[24]

Student Life

Perhaps no one living today can relate completely to the times as they existed in 1883 when the first students of pharmacy began study in Madison. This was a period with minimal noise, light, and air pollution, a time when mechanization and "modern conveniences" were just beginning to emerge. Madison had a population of about 12,000 and the countryside outside of the isthmus was thinly inhabited. The most common means of transportation was walking, although the horse-drawn street car would soon begin operation. For those who could afford it, a horse and carriage could be rented at Kentzler's livery. High-wheeled bicycles were in vogue. Distant communication was mainly by telegraph, since the telephone was a novelty to Madison residents. Lighting was provided by kerosene lamps and by illuminating gas. Running water and bathrooms were not universally available in student residences.[25]

The "Ladies and Gentlemen" of the university were expected to observe the Victorian norm and behave with dignity. Instances of excess were few. Although there was a brewery on State Street with a saloon attached, and similar surrounding institutions, like Tommy Morgan's, drinking in public was done by men only. Intoxication was allegedly infrequent and held in disapproval by student opinion.[26] Men smoked pipes and cigars and a few chewed tobacco, but smoking among the ladies was unknown, at least publicly.[27]

CLASS OF '94

School of Pharmacy

MONDAY EVENING, JUNE 18,

NORTH HALL.

Program

Mandolina Dance, - - - Donigan
Messrs. McCARD and DILLON.

Recitation, "Prior to Miss Belle's Appearance." ——
Miss MARIE MILLER,

ADDRESS,
Mr. JOHN A. DADD.

La Ballerina, - - - - Voth
Messrs. McCARD and DILLON.

Reception

A program and reception honoring the graduating students has been an annual highlight. In 1894 a class of 12 students was addressed by a Milwaukee pharmacist who had given influential support to the developing pharmacy program.

Although rapid changes in transportation, communication and general living conditions occurred during the 1880s and 1890s, social life remained on a relatively even course throughout the late nineteenth century. Literary society meetings, evenings at the Burrows Opera House, class excursions by sleigh or hay wagon to the surrounding countryside, musical entertainment provided by the students, dances, whist and other card games, and social calls were popular forms of extracurricular diversion. "Eating clubs" were consistently popular, while social fraternities and sororities grew to strength in the 1890s. For many of the men, leisure time was filled with hunting and fishing in and around the lakes of Madison. Pharmacy students socialized at meetings of their Pharmaceutical Society and at extemporaneous outings arranged by smaller groups.[28]

One revolutionary change in social life of the late nineteenth century was the rise in popularity of intercollegiate athletics. In 1881, the University Athletic Organization was formed, and Wisconsin joined the Northwestern College League that was organized for baseball. Other sports came to the fore during the 1890s. Although football had been played earlier, it was from 1890 on that UW established a season schedule for a varsity team. By the early 1900s, it is said, the major interest of the students was athletics.[29]

Hazing, the annual fall practice of harassment of freshmen by sophomores, became popular at Wisconsin in the 1870s. Freshmen were made to submit to many indignities. They had to dance, sing, and otherwise entertain their superiors. Their heads were held under a pump, they were thrown in the lake, they were bound and gagged and fined for being "conspicuous." However much the faculty and administration abhorred the practice, they could not halt it. Sometimes the Madison police and court system became involved, but they also were incapable of bringing hazing to an end. Hazing continued in one form or other until the end of World War II and was the source of much amusement among sophomores and animosity among freshmen.[30]

After the turn of the century, changes occurred in almost every decade to alter student extracurricular life. Technological advances brought to students and the general population alike an explosion of new activities. Obvious examples are the development of the automobile, telephone, radio, stereo hi-fi, movies, television, computer and readily available air travel. All have influenced the things students do for enjoyment and entertainment.

Many fads have come and gone. Goldfish swallowing, flagpole sitting, marathon dancing, phone-booth crowding, panty raids, and streak-

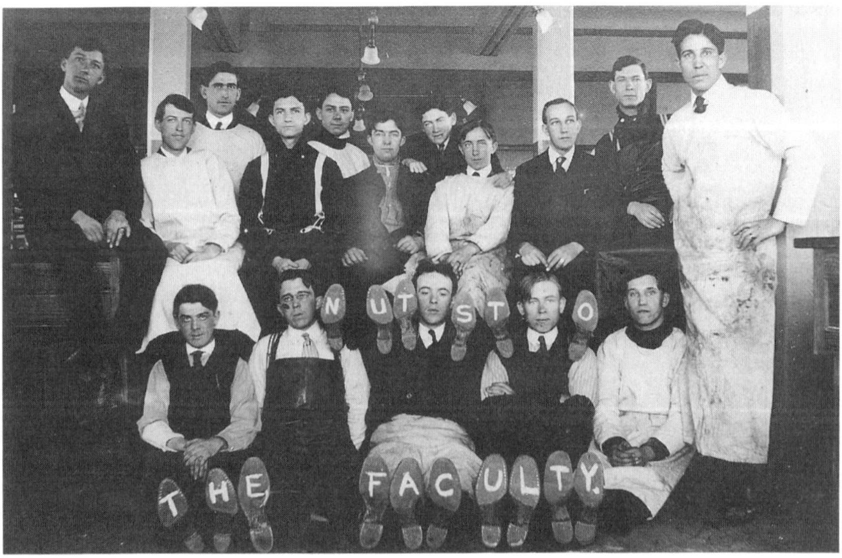

Resourceful students managed to avoid seeming overly respectful of faculty. The pharmacy class of 1903 here makes the point photographically.

ing on Bascom Hill have all been fancies and diversions. However uninterested students sometimes seem in the classroom, they have always been innovative in the pursuit of fun.[31]

While the public may look askance at such student diversions, the University itself has not been immune from criticism of some non-curricular events, real or imagined. In the 1880s, some considered the University a "godless" institution for discontinuing voluntary chapel exercises.[32] Viewing campus laxities with alarm in 1907, the state legislature prohibited the sale of liquor by the drink within 3,200 feet of a main building and condemned students for plans to hold a regatta on Lake Mendota on Memorial Day.[33] Since the end of World War I, some conservatives have persistently thought the Madison campus to be a "breeding ground for political enemies." In the 1930s, the formation of a socialist organization, the Student League for Industrial Democracy, was one factor which prompted outcries against presumed communist tendencies.[34] Few pharmacy students were apparently involved in left-wing organizations, even in the 1930s. The ferment of attitudinal change among students found its most dramatic expression three decades later.[35]

Of the changes in student life at Wisconsin over the past one hundred years, none has been as sweeping as those of the late 1960s. The explosiveness of events in those years overshadowed a more gradual and less dramatic erosion of traditional attitudes ever since World War II.

The sudden influx of war veterans—not only at Wisconsin, but on campuses across the nation—in itself heralded change. Sponsored by the G.I. Bill of Rights, eager to learn, and soberly determined, the student war veteran wanted little to do with traditional schoolboy activities. For the most part, he was interested in progressing through school to a good job and a home in the suburbs, all at the expense of folly. Hazing became a dying custom as veterans, refusing to participate, led the fight against forms of harassment.[36]

At the same time, the campus-wide Student Board of the Wisconsin Student Association (WSA) began considering ways to eliminate compulsory ROTC, opposed a Regent decision not to grant tenure to a popular professor, continued efforts to end racial and religious discrimination, and attempted generally to extend student influence on many fronts, including representation on faculty committees. The Board also started, in 1949, student evaluation of faculty and courses.[37]

The students of the 1950s have been characterized as the "silent generation"[38] because of dwindling participation in student government and apparent preoccupation with athletic events and "panty raids." However, at Wisconsin during this period, many students continued to press for

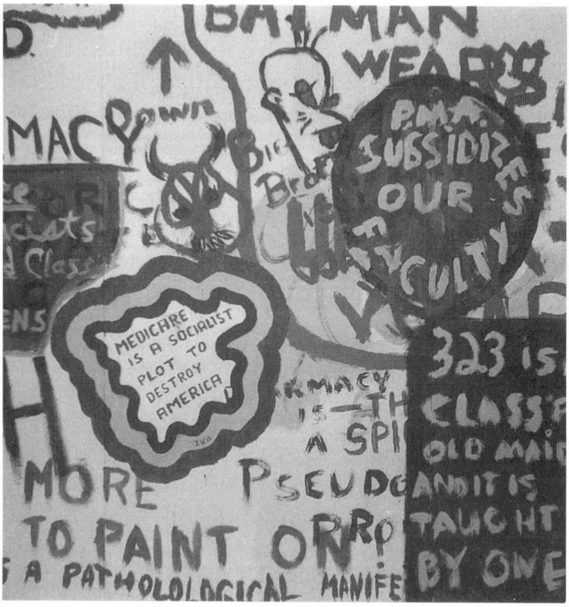
WEAR
P.M.A.
SUBSIDIZES
OUR
CULTY
MEDICARE IS A SOCIALIST PLOT TO DESTROY AMERICA
323 IS
CLASS
OLD MAI
AND IT IS
TAUGHT
BY ONE
A SPI
MORE
PSEUDO
TO PAINT ON
A PATHOLOLOGICAL MANIFE

The rising fad for graffiti and for protest in the late 1960s did not leave pharmacy students entirely untouched.

more freedom, to consider the impact on their activities of UW's imposition of *in loco parentis*, and to express concern about social injustices. In 1953–54, the Associated Women Students began a campaign to extend women's hours and liberalize chaperonage requirements.[39] By 1958, the issue of compulsory ROTC had grown nationwide, and continuous student pressure at Wisconsin resulted in a faculty ruling to abolish it for a two-year trial period. The modern movement for black civil rights—which began with a school desegregation ruling by the U.S. Supreme Court in 1954 and continued with relatively modest skirmishes in the south during the late 1950s—was supported in Madison by a student rally on the library mall and a silent march to the Capitol.[40] A ruling by the Madison faculty in 1960 that unmarried students 21 years of age could live in apartments and could be visited there by members of the opposite sex prompted a more determined student move to end *in loco parentis*.[41]

The spark that lit the biggest blaze in students in the 1960s was the issue of U.S. participation in the Vietnam war, but many other issues came to a head at the same time. Among these were equality for women and minorities, establishment of a department of Afro-American Studies, abolition of on-campus ROTC, the military draft and university relations with the Department of Defense, the legalization of marijuana, and the distribution of birth control information and pills by the Student Health Service. Immediate changes in the status quo were demanded. Demonstrations were sometimes followed by riots and conflict with the National Guard or Madison police. In all, the period between spring 1967 and fall 1970 marked increasing hostility between students and the authorities of the University, city, and state.[42]

Then the bomb went off. An explosion in the middle of the night on August 24, 1970, intended to destroy the Army Math Research Center in Sterling Hall, seriously damaged the adjacent School of Pharmacy; and in the Department of Physics killed one post-doctoral researcher, wasted years of research data, and resulted in the demise of serious student confrontations in Madison as well as across the nation.[43]

The strength of the student revolts of the late 1960s can be sensed from the following facts about students of the 1990s: 1) Students have complete control over their private lives as a result of the discontinuation of *in loco parentis* by the University. 2) The student population consists of approximately proportionate representation by women and minorities. 3) Student representatives are appointed to almost every University committee. 4) Student organizations have been unleashed from faculty control and are, for the most part, free to handle their own affairs.

Student Organizations

Regardless of participation in other activities, events, and organizations on campus, pharmacy students have, from the beginning, organized activities of their own in the School. Student professional organizations have helped establish and maintain an esprit de corps, stimulated companionship among individuals with similar goals, and inculcated professional matters that are not amenable to the formal classroom.

In the early years of the School, organizational life took on special significance because pharmacy students did not participate in most campus-wide activities and organizations. Reportedly many "Hill students,"[44] looked down on the "pharmics" who did not have a degree program (see Chapter 3). To the extent such attitudes prevailed, it probably intensified a sense of purpose in the first internal student organization of the School.[45]

The first pharmacy organization, probably conceived and instituted by Power, was the Pharmaceutical Association of the University of Wisconsin, formed on October 20, 1883. It was reorganized in the fall of 1884 as the Pharmaceutical Society of the University of Wisconsin and continued as such almost to the end of the century.[46]

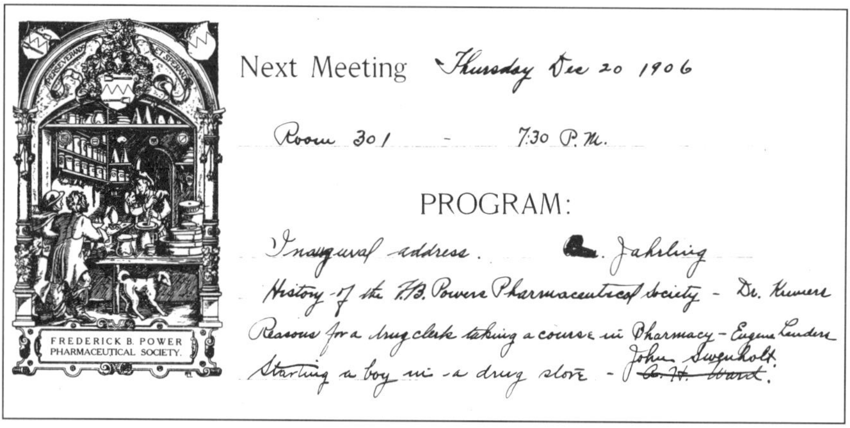

The earliest student organization of the School of Pharmacy announces a meeting. Records of the Society survive in the 710-drawer Edward Kremers Reference Files of the Library.

There are many similarities between the early pharmaceutical organization and the literary societies like Athenaean, Hesperian and Castalia that were started earlier on the Madison campus. The meetings stimulated the extracurricular intellectual and professional life of the students, and they were also intended to be social events. At weekly meetings strict parliamentary practice was emphasized. The organizations elected a censor and assistant censor whose job it was "to note down and impose proper fines upon all members guilty of improper behavior." A critic was also appointed to comment upon the program as presented by students.[47]

At the Pharmaceutical Society meetings, a debate was an integral part and students were selected for participation a week in advance. Topics for debate before the society invariably related to issues in vogue in pharmacy practice of the day. Some of these were: "Should druggists be compelled to pay a government license for selling liquors for medicinal purposes"? "Should druggists make a practice of counter prescribing"? "Should physicians specify special manufacturers names in writing prescriptions"? "Resolved, that lady pharmacists are a success," and "Resolved, that the sale of patent medicines should be discouraged by pharmacists."

Quiz sessions were held during the Society's meetings, at which students were selected at random to answer questions largely pertaining to didactic material presented in the classroom. Student-organized practical demonstrations in chemistry or dispensing were presented and drug displays were made available for viewing during recess.

A musical program was presented at each meeting, usually by pharmacy students themselves (although on at least one occasion, the University glee club was invited to sing). Part of the membership dues went for the rental of Mrs. Prescott's organ and, beyond that, each participant was required to supply his own instrument. In 1894, the society had its own quartet and orchestra.[48]

The roll was called twice during each meeting, at the beginning and following the recess. Members were required to present a written excuse for each absence or be expelled from the organization. Ladies were only required to take part and be present at the quiz session.[49]

Kremers viewed the supplying of practical instruction as one of the main purposes of the Pharmaceutical Society. With the institution of a Department of Practical Pharmacy in the School, interest in the Society began to decline. By 1897, the organization ceased to function for lack of members, and, along with its demise, School spirit seemed to lag.[50]

At the turn of the century, several events contributed to a return of university spirit among pharmacy students. The institution of the four-year, B.Sc. degree program and extension of the pharmacy course over the entire academic year were major factors in gaining a better campus-wide status. Pharmacy students participated in erecting the Students' Boat House and met with the "Hill students" and voted with them in class affairs for the first time. In 1900, one pharmacy student was given representation on the Badger Board and the senior class was given a position on the commencement program. Equally important, school spirit was said to have been boosted by the establishment of Phi Chi Fraternity (re-named Phi Delta Chi, 1909) and by student involvement in publication of the book, *The Badger Pharmacist*.[51]

Delta Chapter of Phi Chi Fraternity was organized at Madison on February 12, 1900, with nine charter members.[52] It began at the University of Michigan in 1883 and by 1909 had grown to include 14 chapters in pharmacy schools in the U.S.A. At Wisconsin, Phi Chi did not last beyond 1903, but was reactivated in 1971 as Delta Chapter of Phi Delta Chi Fraternity. Little is known about the early endeavors of this organization in Madison. Although a professional group, Phi Chi presumably also served the social appetites of its members, as did most of the so-called secret societies on campus during this period.[53] Many of its members contributed to the publication of *The Badger Pharmacist* and it has served as a catalyst in other school activities as well.

The Badger Pharmacist of 1900 was "published in the interests of pharmacy in Wisconsin by the students of the School of Pharmacy of the State University."[54] The book consists of chapters relating to the historical development of pharmacy in Wisconsin and was claimed to be the first attempt of this kind in any state.[55] In addition to historical accounts of pharmaceutical associations of Wisconsin, the state board, legislation, and education, the book contains a biographical sketch (some including pictures) for every graduate of the school from 1883 through 1900. It was widely publicized in pharmaceutical journals and aroused a great deal of interest among pharmacists in the state and elsewhere.[56] However, it was not financially successful and Kremers, who probably was the driving force in its compilation, eventually provided funds to support its publication.[57]

Also around the turn of the century, pharmacy students began making group visits to pharmaceutical manufacturing laboratories. In 1901, the students traveled to Detroit, with a stopover in Chicago. Many trips to drug companies have been made by the students since that time and they are a continuing source of education and amusement.[58]

The dissolution of Phi Chi in 1903 was quickly followed by the beginning of the University of Wisconsin Students Pharmaceutical Association (UWSPhA). This group was formed on October 20, 1904, but, at Kremers' suggestion, changed its name to the F. B. Power Pharmaceutical Society (FBPPhS) on February 2, 1905. This organization was also instigated by Kremers, who had previously seen the need for a student professional organization and the important role it can play in student life.[59]

The object of the UWSPhA and the subsequent FBPPhS was "discussion of questions of pharmaceutical interest and the general advancement of its members in pharmacy and its allied sciences." The organization was patterned after the earlier Pharmaceutical Society and adopted a similar constitution, bylaws and meeting format. It had a sporadic existence from 1904 through 1921 and appeared again in 1934–36. By 1908–09, the meeting format had taken a different appearance, marked by the elimination of musical entertainment and more reliance on outside speakers from among the faculty and pharmacists in the community.[60]

On December 6, 1919, Beta Psi Chapter of Kappa Psi Fraternity was formed at Madison.[61] For several years after the inactivation of the FBPPhS in 1921, Kappa Psi was the only professional pharmacy organization on campus and therefore served as the nucleus for extracurricular activities. However, two factors tended to detract from its role as a pharmacy organization. First, it was an organization to which both pharmacy and medical students could belong. While this helped establish and improve relations between the two professions, it split the allegiance of the group and lessened any control which pharmacy might have hoped to gain in the organization. Second, by the time Kappa Psi was begun at Madison, pharmacy students had become better integrated into campus-wide organizations and activities, which tended to dilute their commitment to pharmacy-related extracurricular affairs.[62]

Kappa Psi did not long remain the only pharmacy organization on campus. The period just after World War I was one of continuing interest in pharmacy students and their organizations. Two movements are of special interest to Wisconsin. One was the drive to form an honorary pharmacy organization along the lines of those existing for students in other professions; the other was to create a professional organization for women pharmacy students.

Out of the first of these emerged the Rho Chi Society. In large measure, it grew out of a local honorary pharmaceutical society at the University of Michigan known as the Aristolochite Society, which was formed in 1908. The development of a national honorary society for pharmacy was suggested by Rufus A. Lyman of Nebraska in 1917, and the nucleus for that expansion was chartered in the state of Michigan as the Rho Chi Society on May 19, 1922. Eta Chapter of Rho Chi was established at Wisconsin in June of 1925.[63]

The recommendation to start a national pharmaceutical sorority also came from Lyman, in 1918. The first of these to appear was Lambda Kappa Sigma. Subsequently, Kappa Epsilon was organized and chartered

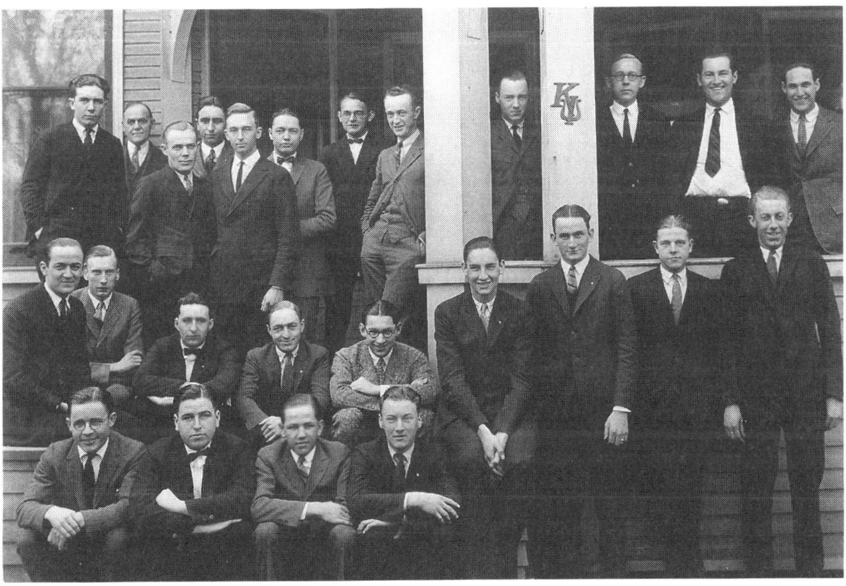

A professional fraternity or sorority has been an important part of social life for many students. Among these Kappa Psi members of 1920–21 was Arthur H. Uhl (front, second from left), who would become the third Director of the School of Pharmacy.

at Wisconsin as Zeta Chapter on April 21, 1926. A precursor to Kappa Epsilon at Wisconsin, known as the Daughters of Aesculapius, had begun the year before with similar purposes and members.[64]

Hence, in the late 1920s, three different organizations for pharmacy students coexisted at Wisconsin. It was a time of relative prosperity, and multiple student organizations would seem to fit in the so-called Era of Excess. However, there was little overlap in membership between these organizations, with two of them excluding the opposite sex.[65]

At the 1928 annual meeting of the American Pharmaceutical Association (APhA), the Committee on Activities of Students and Alumni recommended that a study be made of the feasibility of starting student branches. There was a general feeling on the committee that pharmacists often were insensitive to the value of pharmacy organizations and that there was a need to instill greater pride and loyalty in the profession. It was further felt that the university was the best place to start, since most states by this time had legislated that a pharmacy degree from an accredited school be a prerequisite to licensure.[66] The APhA officially approved the formation of student branches in schools of pharmacy at the 1931 meeting.[67]

Students at Wisconsin made application for a student branch in 1932. This was the sixth such group from schools in the U.S.A. to petition for branch status in the APhA.[68]

The previous year, the WPhA, following the APhA lead, revised its constitution to provide for student membership.[69] An organizational component was not intended and membership in the APhA student branch was not prerequisite for joining WPhA. There is no evidence to indicate that the UW student branch moved at this time to affiliate in any official way with WPhA or to require its members to join WPhA.

Initially, APhA required the student branches to hold two meetings per year and publish their proceedings in the APhA journal.[70] The branch at UW made only one published report, in 1933, implying a lack of extensive interest in the organization. Yet, this organization had been presented with the Beal Organization Award by WPhA in 1932.[71] The branch apparently took an active part in preparations for the national meeting of the APhA that was held in Madison in 1933.[72] Soon thereafter it ceased to exist.

In 1934, the F. B. Power Pharmaceutical Society was revived once again through Kremers' efforts. Although intended to supplement the regular pharmacy curriculum in the tradition of the precursor organization, the meeting format took on a new appearance. Each meeting had a different focus and the speakers (students, faculty, and/or other invited guests) gave scientific talks revolving around the theme of the meeting. The society conducted little business besides the election of officers and the earlier social atmosphere was, for the most part, missing. Reintroduction of a musical program into the meeting format failed to revitalize the organization and it succumbed in 1936.[73]

Just as the depression years were economically difficult for the nation as a whole, substantial hardship was imposed as well on student organizations. Most had become inactive by the late 1930s.[74] Participation in organizations waned as many students found it necessary to work after classes and on weekends to support their existence at the university. The most menial of jobs were eagerly filled by students.[75]

Perhaps in response to the decline in organizational participation, a new student society was begun in 1937. This became known as the Mortar and Pestle Pharmacy Student Organization. It was formed "to promote good fellowship among the members of the faculty and the members of the student body, promote projects in extra-curricular education, inspire a cooperative spirit in all endeavors and occupations, and to develop a friendly way of life among the pharmacy students at the University of Wisconsin." It was further proclaimed that the objectives would "be accomplished by an organized program of social activities during the school year." To this end, the society sponsored parties, an all-pharmacy scavenger hunt, and trips to drug companies. Membership was open to faculty, alumni and all pharmacy students. Apparently there were no meetings of the general membership, but a newsletter, entitled "Mortar and Pestle," was published monthly. This organization had some early success in stimulating student participation, but did not survive beyond the 1938–39 school year.[76]

As a prelude to the 50th-anniversary meeting of the WPhA at Madison in 1930, Kremers began publication of a journal devoted to the history of pharmacy, the first periodical of the kind in America. The title *Badger Pharmacist* was resurrected from the earlier book of the same title, considered to be the forerunner of this publication. The first five issues were published by WPhA, but the remaining issues (through No. 31, 1941) were sponsored by Eta chapter of Rho Chi.[77]

A move to revive the student branch of the APhA was begun in the fall of 1941. The newly formed organization emerged in early 1942 with a revised constitution and new spirit. The student branch of the APhA was also designated as a student branch of the WPhA. This organization, known as the University of Wisconsin Pharmaceutical Society (UWPhS), was the first student branch of the APhA to become officially affiliated with a state pharmaceutical association.[78]

The decline in the number of students during World War II brought also a decrease in activities of the surviving pharmacy organizations. Rho Chi and UWPhS were the only functioning groups during this period, and even the latter ceased to exist in the later stages of the war.[79]

Revival of UWPhS, Kappa Epsilon and Kappa Psi along with changes in student numbers and attitudes after the war began a new era in organized pharmacy student activities.[80] Before the war, meetings and functions of the organizations were exclusively designed to provide information and services to the membership. After the war, organizational activities became more and more community-oriented. At the same time, they provided opportunities for members to gain practical experience in public relations and service. These changes occurred slowly, and it was not until the 1970s that the new style fully developed.

Meanwhile, organizational activities picked up steam, initiated at first by the war veterans. To their lot fell much of the task of rebuilding organizations that had become defunct during the war. Perhaps typifying the times were activities of UWPhS, to which all students were eligible for membership. This group debated the proposed "five-year curriculum", recommended that students have representation on certain faculty committees, created a liaison with WPhA and a public relations committee, were represented at regional meetings of student branches of APhA, discussed the desirability of limiting the number of new pharmacists by controlling enrollment, and competed in contests to create window displays for National Pharmacy Week. The organizational activities probably were influenced by some similar activities of the Wisconsin Student Association in the late 1940s.[81]

Students could volunteer for military drill as early as 1862, and it became compulsory four years later. Although military training sparked occasional controversy, a student referendum in 1927 soundly defeated a proposal to abolish ROTC on campus. In 1948, Wisconsin became one of the first four universities in the U.S.A. to activate a pharmacy ROTC unit. This consisted of a progressive four-year course of military instruction to be taken at the same time as the pharmacy curriculum and with the intent of providing officers with a pharmacy background, who eventually would serve in the Medical Service Corps. The first two years was called the "Basic Pharmaceutical Military Science Course," a prelude to the two-year advanced course. Although this was not, strictly speaking, a pharmacy organization, it did bring with it a common identity and spirit among students participating. By 1956, pharmacy ROTC was dissolved and pharmacy students desiring military training were placed in the Army Medical

Service Corps ROTC. This ceased to function in 1962 at a time when ROTC was becoming less popular on campus.[82]

Many activities of the 1950s could be cited to support the notion that many pharmacy students had more than a casual interest in their professional organizations, thus generating group activities and a spirit of cooperation. Many meetings, colloquies and parties were cosponsored by two or more of the pharmacy organizations. When Pharmacy Week was observed at the School in the fall of 1950, all of the organizations participated. Rho Chi initiated its annual Kremers Memorial Lecture as part of the festivities. Other student projects consisted of displays featuring heart information and promotion of National Pharmacy Week.[83]

In 1951, UWPhS aided the Dane County pharmacists and physicians in distributing detection kits to local pharmacies in conjunction with the Diabetes Detection Drive. For several years beginning in 1953, the organization sponsored a Christmas party for children at Morningside Sanitarium. These may be the first recorded community-oriented functions of a pharmacy organization at the University.[84]

On several occasions during the 1950s, students from other pharmacy schools were drawn to Madison to formally interact with local students.

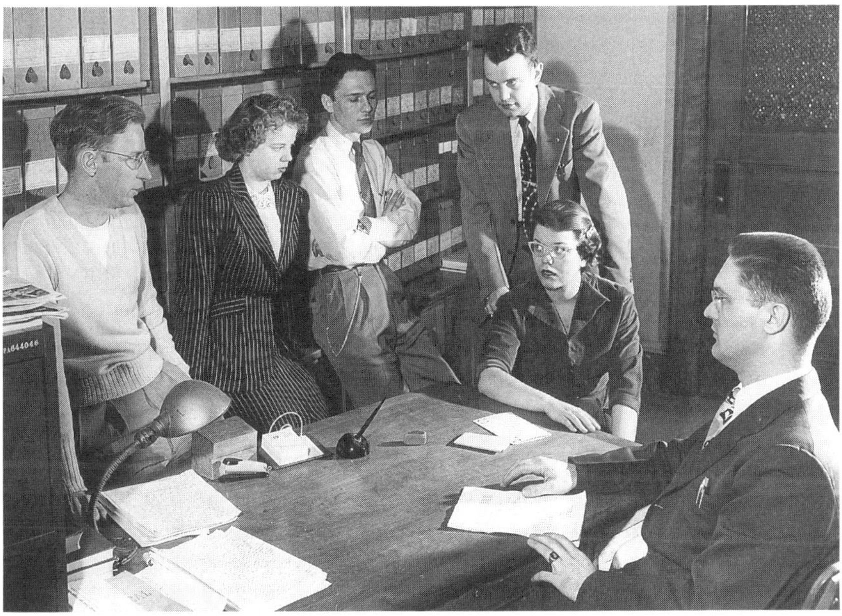

Personal counseling and acquaintanceship between a faculty member and undergraduates flourished when the School was much smaller than it is today. Here Professor Joseph Swintosky confers with a group in his office, about 1950.

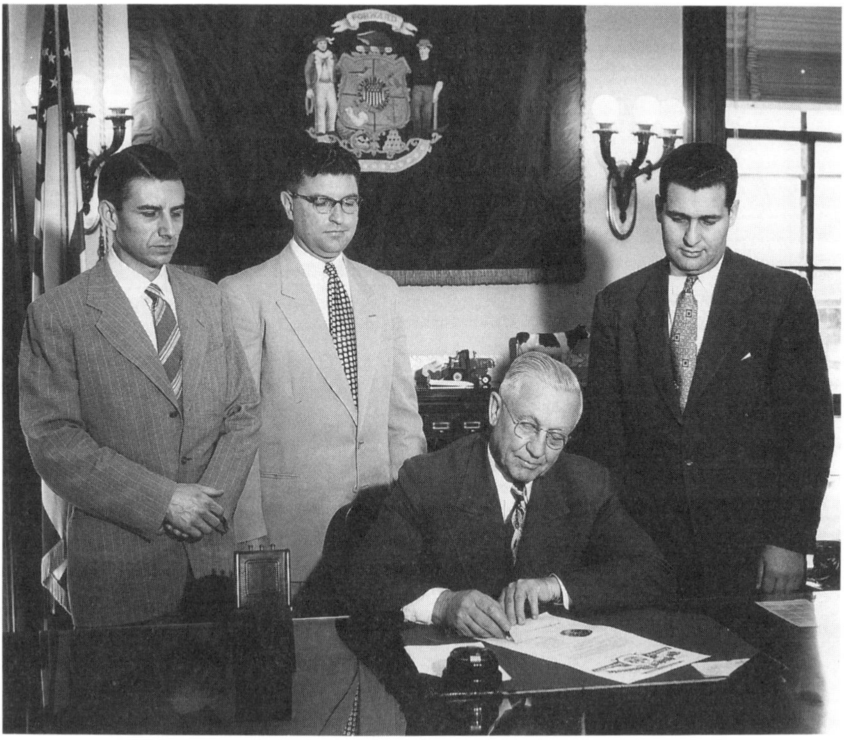

Among the School's distinguished alumni, only one has been Governor of the state, the Wisconsin pharmacist Oscar Rennebohm. In this "photo opportunity" of 1950 the Governor is signing a proclamation, flanked by three UW graduate students: (l. to r.) Glenn Sonnedecker, later a faculty member and the Director of the American Institute of the History of Pharmacy; Leslie M. Lueck, later Vice President for Quality Control and Government Regulations, Parke, Davis and Co.; and William S. Apple, later Executive Director, American Pharmaceutical Association.

UWPhS hosted the Region IV meeting of student branches of the APhA in 1950 and 1956. In 1957, the national meeting of Kappa Epsilon was held in Madison.[85]

By the late 1950s, growing displeasure with the control exerted over their activities by the faculty intensified awareness among students that they had no formal line of communication with the faculty. To provide a voice for the student body, the first Student Council in the School was formed in 1957. There are few recorded activities of the early Council, and meetings appear to have been called infrequently to air problems of interest to the student body.[86]

Cooperative publishing by pharmacy students in the post-war period began in 1945 when reports of school and organizational activities were published in the WPhA's *Wisconsin Druggist*. Although these reports underwent several format changes, continuing into the late 1960s, they conveyed University news items of interest to the students, faculty and pharmacists of the state.[87]

In 1963, a different publishing effort was begun by pharmacy students. It was a periodical titled *Mortar and Quill* and intended as a forum for students regarding professional matters. In addition, *Mortar and Quill* contained news about the activities of each of the School's pharmacy organizations.[88]

In the late 1960s, *Mortar and Quill* began to publish articles of a non-pharmaceutical nature. This change in publication policy can be viewed as part of the campus-wide movement by students to focus attention on national political issues. The mood among pharmacy students, as seen through the *Mortar and Quill*, tended to mirror that which was then sweeping the campus, although it arrived later and was less intensely expressed than it often was elsewhere at UW.[89]

For the most part, pharmacy students were of a conservative bent and the professional organizations continued to function during this period. At its peak the emotional charge that pervaded the campus precipitated protest meetings of the student body and galvanized many pharmacy students into taking a stand on Vietnam and other issues. These events of the late 1960s had an impact on pharmacy students, their lives and their organizational activities. When the UW relinquished the responsibility of *in loco parentis* and discontinued the Office of Student Organization Advisors on campus, students gained new freedoms and enough independence from faculty dominance to chart their own courses.

On March 20, 1971, Delta Chapter of Phi Delta Chi Fraternity was reactivated at Madison. One of the reasons given for reactivation was to help enhance the students' professional spirit.[90] In keeping with this expectation, a major activity of Phi Delta Chi in the 1970s was the establishment of an information program about venereal diseases.[91] Another motivation of the organizers was to mend the broken tradition of Phi Delta Chi at UW and give male students a fraternal alternative to Kappa Psi.

In the late 1970s and early 1980s, a new dimension was added to three of the pharmacy organizations. Kappa Epsilon, Kappa Psi and Phi Delta Chi became coeducational fraternities. This was partly in response to HEW Title IX Guidelines requiring all student organizations, except social fraternities and sororities, to admit both sexes; but the readiness with which it was brought about at Wisconsin testifies to the commitment to coeducation by the students.[92]

During the same period, most of the School's pharmacy organizations also became committed to new activities, especially community-oriented

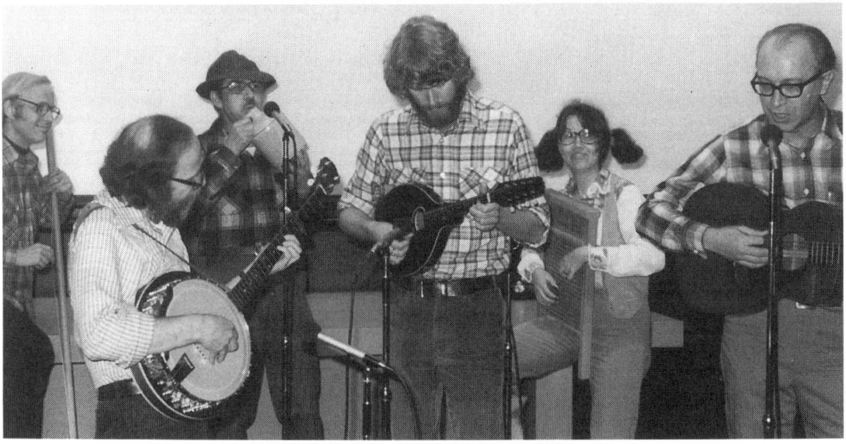

Student social events in the 1970s occasionally featured the Henderson-Hasselbalch String Band. The stellar faculty performers (l. to r.) are Daniel Rich (bass), Kenneth Connors (banjo), Glenn Sonnedecker (jug), Ronald Jasensky (mandolin), Charlotte Anderson-Smith (washboard), and Joseph Robinson (guitar). The group, with some new performers, is still rendering (rending?) bluegrass at School functions.

service projects, the sum of which articulated with changes permeating the previous postwar decades.

Kappa Epsilon became involved in conducting a poison-prevention puppet show in cooperation with the Auxiliary of the WPhA and presenting programs such as "Cold Remedies" and "Antacids" to local groups. They also sponsored Halloween parties for patients at Children's Hospital at UW, entertained residents of a convalescent center in Madison and donated proceeds from hot-dog sales to charitable organizations.[93]

Kappa Psi presented drug-abuse education programs in Madison's primary and secondary schools, sponsored an annual Halloween party (donating the profits to UNICEF), and organized a blood drive in the School. Members also were active in diabetes screening in the Madison area, performed drug audits concerning generic substitution and presented a slide program entitled "Your Future in Pharmacy" to high school and pre-pharmacy classes in Madison and Milwaukee.[94]

In addition to its participation in venereal disease informational services, Phi Delta Chi developed several public education programs for presentation to community groups. Some of the topics were "Poisoning Prevention," "Arthritis," "Alcoholism," and "What is a Drug and How does it Work?". In the fall of 1981, Delta chapter received a Certificate of Recognition from the American Cancer Society for its activities as campus-wide coordinator for the Great American Smokeout.[95]

UWPhS (and SAPhA) actively promoted Pharmacy Week, Poison Prevention Week, the Great American Smokeout, and drug information to the public. In the late 1970s, SAPhA instituted a program for blood-pressure screening, a slide presentation on mental depression, a geriatric screening committee, active public relations and legislative committees and an annual Drug Fair.[96]

The ethos pervading the pharmacy organizations in recent times echoes the heightened social consciousness of students begun in the 1960s.

Student Awards

Many awards have been given to pharmacy students over the years. Several have come from drug companies and pharmacy organizations to honor individuals with leadership capabilities. Other awards have consisted of funds for especially needy students in support of their university education. However, none have more significance in a university than those given for academic achievement.

In 1884, WPhA members voted unanimously to award a gold medal to the student with the highest general average on the comprehensive final examination. In 1885, the gold medal presented to Henry G. Ruenzel of Milwaukee was the first scholastic achievement award given to a pharmacy student at UW.[97]

The award for academic excellence with the longest tradition is that of the Rho Chi Society (Eta chapter), a recognition of the first-year pharmacy student with the highest scholastic achievement. For recipients of this award, established in 1941, see *Appendix 4e*. The first recipient was Floyd P. Hallett.[98]

Beginning in 1966, Eli Lilly and Company made available an award to be presented to the graduating senior with the highest cumulative grade-point average (GPA). For recipients of this award, see *Appendix 4f.* The first was Patricia Williams.[99]

The David Perlman Scholarship Award, named in recognition of a former Dean of the School, has been presented by Phi Delta Chi since 1979. It is given to each member of Delta chapter having a GPA of 3.5 or above during the first five semesters in The School of Pharmacy.[100]

In 1937 and 1948, Zeta chapter of Kappa Epsilon was the winner of a traveling Chapter Scholarship Trophy awarded to the chapter having the highest GPA in the largest number of years over a ten-year period. In 1967, they were again distinguished by recording the highest GPA of all Kappa Epsilon chapters.[101]

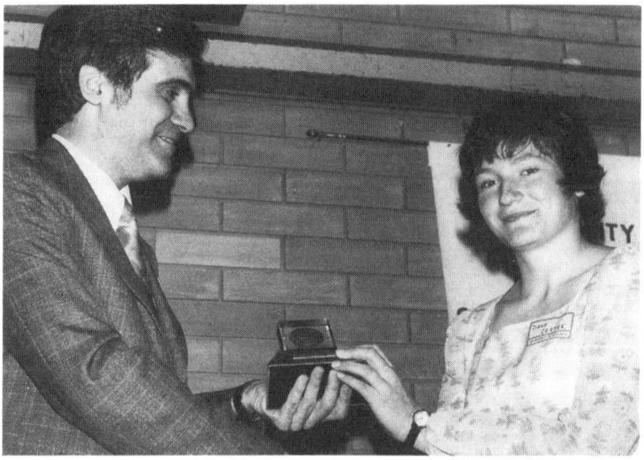

Student awards are presented at the traditional graduation-day luncheon for seniors, parents, and faculty. Dean George Zografi is shown, in 1976, presenting the award for highest cumulative grade-point average to Diane Cramer.

Conclusion

The UW School of Pharmacy exists for its students; and the students of every generation helped determine the development and spirit of the institution during its first century. The student activities here recorded did not, of course, occur in isolation from the milieu of the University at large. Interactions with the organizations, faculty, other students on campus, students on other campuses, and with non-students all have had their evolutionary consequences. However, able and eager participation has had a pivotal role in extracurricular contributions to the life of the School and the memories of alumni.

Notes and References

1. F. C. Young, "On the Importance of Students, 1949–1974," *in The University of Wisconsin; One Hundred and Twenty-Five Years*, A. G. Bogue and R. Taylor, eds., (Madison, 1975), 133.
2. All enrollment figures were compiled by Dr. Gregory J. Higby from the following sources: Pharmacy enrollment figures were obtained from: University of Wisconsin Catalogues and School of Pharmacy Bulletins (1883–1943); University phone directories (women) and School of Pharmacy records, Edward Kremers Reference Files (men) (1943–1946); First Semester enrollment figures, UW Archives (1947–1952); "Undergraduate Enrollment," document from U.W. Registrar's Office (1952–1958, 1978–1981); Annual enrollment figures from *Am. J. Pharm. Ed.* (1959–1978). Total U.W. enrollment figures were obtained from: University Catalogues (1883–1967 except 1940–41, 1943–46); "University of Wisconsin Enrollments (Madison Campus)," document from

"Enrollment" folder in Archives, vertical subject file (1940–41, 1943–46); *Opening Fall Enrollment in Higher Education,* (1967–1976); *Collegiate Enrollment in the United States,* (1976–1981). Pharmacy enrollment figures do not reflect the number of students on the Milwaukee campus.

3. E. Kremers, Report of Committee on School of Pharmacy of WPhA, 12, in KRF, C31(a)I.
4. It was the opinion of the Dean of Pharmacy at Minnesota that the Spanish War was over before it could have a significant impact on enrollment. Charles V. Netz, *History of the University of Minnesota College of Pharmacy, 1892 1970,* (Minneapolis, 1971), 20.
5. J. J. Abel, C. L. Alsberg, R. F. Bacon, F. R. Eldred, R. Hunt, T. B. Johnson, J. Stieglitz, F. O. Taylor and C. H. Herty, *The Future Independence and Progress of American Medicine in the Age of Chemistry. A Report,* (New York, 1923), 7–14; Merle Curti and Vernon Carstensen, *The University of Wisconsin; A History 1848–1925,* (Madison, 1949), I, 306; *JWPhA,* 1 (1920): No. 3, 6.
6. List of SATC pharmacy students in KRF, C31(a)I.
7. Interview with Lawrence F. Madland, April 13, 1981.
8. *Wis. Drugg.,* May, 1941, 10; ibid., July, 1942, 9; ibid., April, 1943, 5; ibid., August, 1943, 11.
9. *Wis. Drugg.,* November, 1945, 15; ibid., July, 1946, 26; ibid., October, 1946, 8.
10. A barracks from Camp McCoy was set up in the woods near Chadbourne Hall for the use of pharmacy students. It was divided into three laboratories and provided with new equipment. *Wis. Drugg.,* January, 1947, 10.
11. Curti and Carstensen, (n. 5), I, 374.
12. *Pharm. Era,* 15 (1896): 468; graduation records were compiled by Gregory J. Higby from the following sources: *Catalogue* (1884–1924); loose-leaf list of graduates and theses (1884–1964) in the F. B. Power Pharmaceutical Library and 4310 Chamberlin Hall (untitled) (1925–1964); document titled "Degrees Conferred," University of Wisconsin Office of the Registrar (1964–1980).
13. Patricia S. Ward, "Hygeia's Sisters: A History of Women in Pharmacy," *Caduceus,* 4(1988): 37–40.
14. Interview, with Eunice Bonow Bardell, April 27, 1981.
15. Ward, (n. 13), 15–17; Nellie Wakeman, "Women in Pharmacy," *J. APhA,* 26 (1937): 560–561. The shortage of females in pharmacy in 1911 created a contest among the male students for a seat beside her in class. The earliest riser for an 8 a.m. class won the distinction. *The Pill,* 2 (1911): 16.
16. W. H. Chafe, *The American Woman: Her Changing Social, Economic and Political Roles, 1920–1970* (Cambridge, 1972), 245–254.
17. Dean A. H. Uhl cautiously outlined reasons for recruiting women into pharmacy during World War II. The major thrust was that women were needed to meet the civilian demand for pharmacists. An attempt was made to assure pharmacists of the state that the recruitment program was intended primarily to function as part of the war effort. The WPhA appointed a special committee to recruit females into pharmacy from among the high school graduates and sponsored an informal reception at the Schroeder Hotel in Milwaukee on September 16, 1943, for all such interested persons. A. H. Uhl, "Why is Pharmacy a Desirable Profession for Women?," *Wis. Drugg.,* June,

1943, 8; A. H. Uhl, untitled, *ibid.*, July, 1943, 10; S. H. Dretzka, "Reception for Girl Pharmacist Prospects. WPhA Special Committee on Women in Pharmacy," *ibid.*, September, 1943, 13.

18. The numbers of female pharmacy students were: 15 in 1942–43, 28 in 1943–44, 25 in 1944–45 and 51 in 1945–46. Compiled by Gregory J. Higby from sources listed in footnote 2.
19. The numbers of female pharmacy students between 1936–37 and 1939–40 averaged 15 per year. The numbers between 1947–48 and 1959–60 averaged 34 per year. In 1954–55, 18 female students were enrolled in the school. Figures compiled by Gregory J. Higby from sources listed in footnote 2.
20. Chafe, *Woman*, (n. 16), 245–254.
21. The growth of the pharmacy female population at Wisconsin paralleled that in other pharmacy schools in the U.S. Female enrollments in all schools of pharmacy in 1965–66 and 1979–80 were 14 and 43%, respectively, while at Wisconsin, the respective percentages were 12 and 40. There was also an expansion of female enrollment in other health professions during a similar period. Between 1971 and 1978, female enrollment increased by 218% in medicine, 832% in dentistry and 317% in veterinary medicine. Also, the percentage of females in the total civilian work force rose from 38.2% in 1970 to 41.6% in 1978. *APhA Task Force: Women in Pharmacy*, (Washington, D.C., 1981), 14. Most females who enrolled in pharmacy in the 1970s were interested primarily in combining a career in pharmacy with a home and family life. K. W. Kirk and M. L. Henderson, "Expectations of Female Pharmacy Students," *J. APhA*, NS15, (1975): 623. Females represented 24.4% of all students on the Madison campus in 1949–50 and 40.4% in 1973–74. C. R. Ruedisili, "Evolving Undergraduate and Graduate Curricula, 1949–74" *In* Bogue and Taylor, (n. 1), 160.
22. D. Perlman, Dean, report to WPhA, *Wis. Pharm.*, May, 1973, 155.
23. In 1932, there were only 330 registered black pharmacists in the country. Up to that time and several years beyond, a principal concern was to have black pharmacists to serve the black community, less concern about total integration. J. J. Mullowney, "What Future Is There for the Negro Pharmacist?," *J. APhA*, 21 (1932): 1188.
24. G. Zografi, "School of Pharmacy Report at the 1976 WPhA Convention," *Wis. Pharm.*, November, 1976, 382; G. Zografi, "School of Pharmacy Annual Report. 1977 WPhA Convention," ibid., December, 1977, 475; University of Wisconsin–Madison Faculty Document 439, May 4, 1981, 10–11.
25. Curti and Carstensen, (n. 5), I, 390–392, 670; *Picturesque University of Wisconsin*, reprinted from Special Numbers of *The Daily Cardinal*, ed. by W. H. Hobbs, March, 1898, 1–2; F. A. Pike, *A Student at Wisconsin Fifty Years Ago*, (Madison, 1935), 10–13, 30, 188; Russell W. Archer, *"Drugs and Medicine, Tobacco and Segars": As Madison Grows, Pharmacy Grows*, (Madison, 1980), 180–188; E. Kremers, "Dr. Power at Wisconsin," *The Badger Pharmacist*, No. 13, 1936, 5–9.
26. Pike, (n. 25), 130–132; Pharmacy students added a touch of their own inclination (or levity) in the University yearbook by sponsoring a page for the "Pharmaceutical Temperance Society" which had "no members" and met "regularly seldom." (*Trochos*, 1885, 148). Drinking of the "brew itself was mostly taboo in faculty circles in which tea was served." Kremers, "Power" (n.

5), 5. By the late 1970s and early 1980s, alcohol abuse by students at UW was considered a serious problem, more so than drug abuse, and the University began offering informational and awareness workshops and distributing pamphlets about alcoholism. *Wisconsin State Journal*, August 16, 1981.

27. According to Kremers, equipment for pharmacy students was very sparse in the early days. In one of the laboratories, the students shared three pipettes. His chagrin for this situation was implied by his statement that "some of my classmates chewed tobacco, some of us did not." Kremers, "Power" (n. 5), 5.

28. Pike, (n. 25), 36, 57, 171, 181, 187; Curti and Carstensen, (n.5), I, 432–433, 665; *Wis. Drugg. Exchange*, 2 (1893): No. 5, 3; One graduate has related his experiences on a hiking trip to the Wisconsin countryside with friends during his student days. E. Kremers Papers, Archives, State Historical Society of Wisconsin, Wis/Mss/NB/Box 9.

29. Pike, (n. 25), 137, 141. The yell U-ra-ra Wis-con-sin was developed in 1884, ibid., 152. Curti and Carstensen, (n. 5), I, 387–389, 572, 697. The decline in popularity of literary societies in the 1890s can, in part, be attributed to the rise in popularity of intercollegiate athletics. Ibid. 433.

30. Many incidents of hazing at Wisconsin have been reported. Ibid., 386–87, 548–555 and Pike, (n. 25), 31–33. In the late 1920s, one pharmacy student was hazed by being thrown into Lake Mendota. He swam for some distance underwater before surfacing unseen beneath a nearby pier and thereby created a great deal of fear in his attackers. Conversation with Clarence Sondern, July 22, 1981.

31. Source materials for fads were C. B. T. Lee, *The Campus Scene, 1900–1970. Changing Styles in Undergraduate Life* (New York, 1970), and Young, (n. 1).

32. Curti and Carstensen, (n. 5), I, 410.

33. Ibid., II, 178.

34. D. Long, "Wisconsin: Changing Styles of Administrative Response," *in* J. Foster and D. Long, *Protest! Student Activism in America*, (New York, 1970), 247.

35. C. B. T. Lee, (n. 31), 63–72.

36. Ibid., (n. 31), 82–87.

37. C. M. McIntyre, "The Influence and Influence Strategies of the Wisconsin Student Association on University Policy Making, 1938–1970," (Ph.D. thesis, University of Wisconsin, 1972), 79, 90, 94, 97.

38. Lee, (n. 31), 88.

39. By 1963, females at Wisconsin were allowed some of the most liberal hours of any campus in the nation and, in the spring of 1968, regulations on hours were totally abolished. McIntyre, (n. 37), 129, 222, 315.

40. The rally on library mall in spring of 1960 was the first Student Senate-supported demonstration at UW. Although the Senate did not formally support the silent march to the Capitol, a precedent was, nevertheless, set by this action. Ibid., 176–177.

41. Ibid., 172–173.

42. Ibid., 291–369; Long, (n. 34), 246–270; J. Ridgeway, *The New Republic*, 157 (1967): No. 19, 8–10; M. W. Miles, *The Radical Probe. The Logic of Student Rebellion*, (New York, 1971), 59–61.

43. The Pharmacy Building, located just across a narrow alley from Sterling Hall, suffered extensive damage. *Wis. Pharm.*, October, 1970, 404.

44. Students attending the University were said to be "on the Hill." *Picturesque University of Wisconsin*, (n. 25), 2.

45. E. Kremers, Report on Fifty Years of Organized Pharmacy Activities in Wisconsin, in KRF; *Proc. WPhA, 1896*, 43.

46. Minutes Book of the Pharmaceutical Society of the University of Wisconsin, in KRF. A letter from H. G. Ruenzel to E. Kremers in KRF indicates that only seniors were allowed to become members at first. Later, it is suggested, the juniors and seniors came together, but later split again. If there was a selective membership in the organization, it is not reflected in the *Wisconsin Badger* yearbook, which lists members from both classes. The object of the Pharmaceutical Association was "the extension of scientific knowledge among its members, and the promotion of all interests relative to their studies." *Trochos*, 1885, 106. The Pharmaceutical Society had as its object "to bring students in Pharmacy together for the purpose of exchanging ideas and discussing the questions relating to Pharmacy that they may be better prepared to meet the requirements of their profession." *Trochos*, 1887, 108.

47. It is not surprising that the pharmacy organization would attempt to emulate the literary societies since the latter were dominant in university student politics and social affairs until the mid–1890s when social fraternities and athletics grew to prominence. Curti and Carstensen, (n. 5), I, 421–438, 665. Members at Pharmaceutical Society meetings were fined or criticized by the Censor for imitating cats, speaking profanities, spitting on the floor, using the word "chestnuts," throwing objects at the President and failing to remove their hats when entering the room. Minutes Book of Society in KRF.

48. *Wis. Drugg. Exchange*, 3, (1894): 86; Edward Kremers Papers, (Wis. Mss. NB), in Archives Division of State Historical Society of Wisconsin.

49. Most of the information was taken from the Minutes Book of the Society in KRF. See also *Wisconsin Druggist Exchange*, 2 (April 1893): 3; ibid., (May 1893): 3; ibid., (November 1893): 2; ibid., 3 (November, 1894): 86; ibid., 5 (1896): 90.

50. *Proc. WPhA*, 1900, 33.

51. Ibid.; *Pharm. Rev.*, 18, (1900): 81 (advertisement).

52. Jack R. Arndt, "The Spirit is Back, Delta Reactivated," *The Communicator*, 60, (1971): No. 3, 6–8; *The Badger Pharmacist*, (Madison, 1900), 141; *Northwest. Drugg.* 1, (1900): No. 4, 16; *Wis. Drugg. Exch.*, 9 (1900): 20.

53. John D. Grabenstein, ed., *Phi Delta Chi: A Tradition of Leaders in Pharmacy* (Athens, GA, (1995), 120–122 concerning the UW chapter. An example of entertainment of the times is given by a Phi Chi dance card in KRF. On Friday evening, December 7, 1900, the fraternity sponsored a dance at Keeley's Hall. Students (and chaperones) danced the waltz and two-step to such tunes as "Wake Up Ma Baby," "Hunky Dory," "Lucy Ducy," "Dusky Dudes" and "Hot Old Time in Rag Town."

54. *The Badger Pharmacist*, (Madison, 1900), 292. This book was most likely initiated and heavily edited by Kremers. *Northwest. Drugg.*, 2 (1901): No. 4, 20.

55. Ibid., iii (Preface).

56. Many letters are on file in KRF attesting to the widespread interest in this publication. See also *Wis. Drugg. Exch.*, 9 (1900): 20; *Northwestr. Drugg.*, 2, (1901): 20; *Pharm. Era*, 1901, February 14, 190; *Pharm. Rev.*, 19, (1901): 13 (advertisement).

57. *The Badger Pharmacist* of 1900 sold for $1 per copy. When, in 1909, the F. B. Power Pharmaceutical Society voted to publish a similar book, it was pointed out at the meeting that the cost of the original edition had been $753, that $453 had been paid by sales and that $300 had been paid by Kremers. There is no mention of the source of the $300, but the loss was apparently sufficient stimulus to deter the students (or, more likely, Kremers) from accomplishing publication of a 1910 edition. Minutes Book of F. B. Power Pharmaceutical Society in KRF.

58. *Wis. Drugg. Exch.*, 10, (1901): 29; *Pharmaceutical Review*, 19, (1901): 29; Pharmacy students had also taken a field trip to Milwaukee the previous year to view factories "in which chemical processes are conducted" and it is possible that this included a visit to Kremers & Urban Co. *Pharm. Rev.*, 18, (1900): 81 (advertisement), *Wis. Drugg. Exch.*, 9, (1900): 46. The records of student visits to several drug companies are incomplete. Trips to Eli Lilly and Company are on record as early as 1920. *J. WPhA*, 1 (1920) No. 3, 13. Written responses to inquiries made by Gregory J. Higby indicate that pharmacy students from UW began making tours of Abbott Laboratories, Chicago, in 1953; The Upjohn Company, Kalamazoo, in 1946, and Parke, Davis & Company, Detroit, before 1933. The records of student visitations in possession of the latter company only date back to 1933, but the trip made from Madison to Detroit in 1901 was for the purpose of visiting this company. Also, in Detroit, the students visited Frederick Stearns and Co. *Pharm. Rev.*, 19, (1901): 85 (advertisement). The response from Kremers & Urban Co. of Milwaukee was that small groups of students (primarily members of Phi Delta Chi) had visited them since 1978, although such field trips probably began earlier. In 1974, The Upjohn Company discontinued receiving students, but instituted an "on campus visitation program." This program was presented in Madison for the first time on December 2, 1981.

59. Minutes Book of the UWSPhA and FBPPhS in KRF; *Wis. Drugg.*, 2 (1904): February, 6.

60. Ibid., see also, *Wis. Drugg.*, 4, (1906): April, 4, Ibid., 4, (1906): November 5 and Ibid., 5, (1907): February, 4.

61. F. H. Eby, *The History of Kappa Psi Pharmaceutical Fraternity, 1879–1966*, (Kappa Psi Pharmaceutical Fraternity, 1967), 64.; *J. WPhA*, 1, (1920): No. 1, 15.

62. At the time the fraternity filed to become a legal corporation, the purposes were stated to be "to conduct a mutual fraternal organization having for its object the mutual education and social advancement of its members and to this end unite in fraternal union persons of good character and sound mental health by conferring upon them certain degrees which shall exemplify industry, sobriety, mutual education and advancement both in the study of medicine and pharmacy-to assist the faculty of colleges, universities, or other educational institutions in which it is, or shall be established, in promoting such studies and in any or every way whatsoever advance their interests." When medicine and pharmacy split in 1924, the new pharmaceutical fraternity became known as Kappa Psi Pharmaceutical Fraternity, retaining much of the

original purposes, but placing more emphasis on participation in pharmacy-related activities. Ibid., 9, 12–13, 125; *Handbook and Pledge Manual of Kappa Psi Pharmaceutical Fraternity, Inc.*, (n.p., 1981), 3. Kappa Psi has been the only pharmacy organization at UW to maintain a house for its members. The houses have been located on Mills Street, near Johnson Street (1920), 115 Ely Place (1921), 106 West Dayton Street (1922), 640 North Frances Street (1923), 211 Langdon Street (1925), 619 Mendota Court (1951) and 615 North Lake Street (1963-present). The latter house was purchased in 1972. *J. WPhA*, 2, (1921): No. 1, 19; ibid., 2, (1921): No. 10, 14; *The Badger Yearbook*, (Madison, 1923), 464; ibid., 1924, 473; *Wis. Drugg.*, February, 1957, 12; *Wis. Pharm.*, March, 1963, 78; ibid., May, 1972, 124; G. J. Albright, "A History of Beta Psi Chapter of Kappa Psi," student ms. essay in KRF.

63. Roy A. Bowers and D. L. Cowen, *The Rho Chi Society, The Development of the Honor Society of American Pharmacy*, 4th ed., (Columbus, OH, 1978), 1; L. F. Dobberke, "The History of the Rho Chi Society of the University of Wisconsin," student ms. essay in the KRF. The object of Rho Chi "has always been to promote the advancement of the pharmaceutical sciences through the encouragement and recognition of sound scholarship." Furthermore, Rho Chi "seeks to promote scholarly fellowship in pharmacy by bringing undergraduate and graduate students, and faculty members together in fraternal and helpful association." It also "seeks to increase the awareness of the ethical and social responsibilities of the profession, and thereby to enhance the prestige of the profession" and "to encourage research in pharmacy." The constitution of Rho Chi states that "The object of the society shall be the promotion of scholarship, friendship, and the recognition of the high attainments in the pharmaceutical sciences." On all points, membership in Rho Chi is one of the highest academic honors that can be given a pharmacy student since members are selected for scholarly achievement. *Rho Chi Society, History, Constitution and Bylaws*, (1977–78 Revision), 2.

64. Kappa Epsilon was formally organized on May 13, 1921 by representatives from the University of Minnesota, University of Nebraska and University of Iowa. E. R. Bonow, "The History of Professional Pharmaceutical Fraternities for Women," *Am. J. Pharm. Ed.*, 18, (1954): 410–413. *Guide to Kappa Epsilon Fraternity*, 2nd ed., (Kappa Epsilon Fraternity, 1979), 8. The original name of the precursor group at UW was reported in pharmaceutical journals as the "Girls' Pharmaceutical Club." *Pharmacal News*, 11, (1926): No. 9, 3. Subsequently, the name was changed, at the suggestion of Kremers, to Daughters of Aesculapius. Scrapbook of Kappa Epsilon, in possession of Zeta chapter, School of Pharmacy. The purposes of Kappa Epsilon are "to unite the women students in pharmacy; to cooperate with the faculties of the colleges where chapters are established; to stimulate in its members a desire for high scholarship; to foster a professional consciousness; and to provide a bond of lasting loyalty, interest and friendship." The objects of the predecessor organization at Wisconsin were "to foster a spirit of fraternalism, unite the women employed in pharmaceutical pursuits for mutual encouragement and assistance, to assist in the advancement of pharmaceutical education and to cooperate with college authorities in the efforts to maintain high social and scholastic standards." *Guide to Kappa Epsilon Fraternity*, 3; *Pharmacal News*, 11, (1926): No. 9, 3.

65. In the early years of Rho Chi, most of the members were graduate students. *Badger Pharm.*, (1931): No. 6, 1. In 1980, a small group of pharmacy students started an organization with the purpose of providing a social alternative to existing organizations and focusing on the nonacademic aspects of student life. Although the name of this new organization, Rho Lo, implied a counter to the high academic standards of Rho Chi, membership was available to all pharmacy students, independent of scholastic achievement. (Conversation with faculty-advisor Paul Bass, February 3, 1982).

66. B. V. Christensen, "Student Branches of American Pharmaceutical Association," *J. APhA*, 19, (1930): 390–393. Prerequisite legislation, a law requiring applicants for the state board examination in pharmacy to be graduates of accredited schools of pharmacy, became effective in Wisconsin on July 28, 1927. *Proc. WPhA, 1927*, 147–153.

67. *J. APhA*, 20, (1931): 810.

68. Wisconsin (*J. APhA*, 21, (1932): 76) was preceded by schools of pharmacy at the University of Pittsburgh (*J. APhA*, 18, (1929): 1059), State College of Washington (*J. APhA*, 20, (1931): 401), State College of South Dakota (*J. APhA*, 20, (1931): 597), Western Reserve (*J. APhA*, 20, (1931): 1130) and University of Florida (*J. APhA*, 21, (1932): 72), in order of published petitions. Actually, there was no published petition from the University of Pittsburgh. The students there had become an "unofficial" student branch before APhA changed its constitution to provide for student branches. Also, the University of North Carolina and University of Washington had earlier organized as "local branches" of APhA, in association with local pharmacists. *Apharmacy Weekly*, 20, (1981): No. 45, 188; *The Pharmacy Student*, 11, (1981): No. 4, 3. Of the early student branches to form before 1940, only the group at Western Reserve was also officially affiliated with a local branch of the APhA. *J. APhA*, 18, (1929): 419–420.

69. *Badger Pharmacist*, (1931): No. 6, 10; *Proc. WPhA, 1931*, 106–107.

70. *J. APhA*, 19, (1930): 1150–1151.

71. *Wis. Drugg.*, July, 1933, 10; ibid., January, 1934, 6. The Beal Organization Prize was established by James H. Beal of Ohio at the Jubilee meeting of the WPhA in 1931. Beal was an invited speaker at the meeting and not only refused to accept a $100 honorarium, but added another $100 to establish a prize to be presented to the local association which could demonstrate "the greatest progress in its organization efforts." *Badger Pharm.*, (1931): No. 6, 13.

72. *J. APhA*, 22, (1933): 358.

73. Attendance at society meetings was required of all students enrolled in Pharmacy 50 and Pharmacy 1. This was in lieu of one class per month in each of these courses. Some meeting themes included "Vehicles in Medicine," "Drug Extraction," "Castor Oil," "New Ointment Bases" and "Cellulose." A different faculty advisor was responsible for helping organize each meeting. Minutes Book of FBPPhS in KRF, C36(f) I-Wisconsin.

74. Kappa Epsilon became inactive in 1939 and had a brief reappearance in 1941. It is presumed to have been inactive in the years 1942–43 and 1943–44 since no officers were listed for this period. P. Bergman and M. Boernke, "History of Zeta Chapter of Kappa Epsilon," student ms. essay in KRF. Kappa Psi became dormant in 1935, was reactivated for a brief period in 1939, but failed again in 1941 due to the war. G. J. Albright, "A History of Beta Psi Chapter of

Kappa Psi," student ms. essay in KRF. No record of officers of Rho Chi is available between 1931–32 and 1938–39 (L. F. Dobberke, student manuscript), but Rho Chi was active during the early and mid–1930s as witnessed by reports of their functions. *Wis. Drugg.*, July, 1934, 38; ibid., April 1935, 19, 30; ibid., February, 1936, 28; *Badger Pharm.*, (1931): No. 6, 1, 8; ibid., (1931): No. 7, 1, 12; ibid., (1936): No. 8, 13; ibid., (1936): No. 12, 15.

75. Conversation with Lawrence Madland of Milwaukee, April, 13, 1981.

76. *Mortar and Pestle*, 1 (1938): No. 1, 1; ibid., No. 2, 1, in KRF.

77. *Badger Pharm.*, (1931): No. 6, 1; ibid., (1936): No. 12, 15; ibid., (1941): No. 31, 11; *Mortar and Pestle*, 1, (1938): No. 2.

78. Minutes Book of UWPhS. *Wisconsin State Journal*, May 5, 1942. When the student branch reorganized in 1942, it actually formed three organizations having similar constitutions. The group was known as the University of Wisconsin Student Branch of the American Pharmaceutical Association, the University of Wisconsin Student Branch of the Wisconsin Pharmaceutical Association and the University of Wisconsin Pharmaceutical Society (UWPhS). The objectives of the three organizations were similar, but that of the latter included "to coordinate the activities of the Student Branch of APhA and WPhA." In 1968, UWPhS adopted a single constitution with a revised objective that "It shall function as and shall be an associate (student) chapter of the American Pharmaceutical Association and of the Wisconsin Pharmaceutical Association." On December 7, 1976, another revised constitution of UWPhS was adopted and the name of the society became the University of Wisconsin Student American Pharmaceutical Association (UWSAPhA) in accordance with that of the national organization. The main object of the group remained "to promote an active interest in the advancement of the profession of pharmacy and pharmaceutical learning and to create a better understanding and fellowship among those persons interested in pharmacy." It continued to be an associate of WPhA. *Constitution of UWPhS, 1942*; *Constitution of UWPhS* (Revised, 1968); *Constitution of UWSAPhA* (Revised, 1976); *Wis. Pharm.*, September, 1976, 292.

79. Minutes Book of UWPhS, KRF, C36(f)I:Wis.

80. Kappa Epsilon was reactivated in 1944–45 (Bergman and Boernke, n.74) and Kappa Psi on November 11, 1949 (Eby, n. 61), 64. UWPhS became active again in 1947. Minutes Book of UWPhS. Rho Chi survived the war, (L. F. Dobberke, student manuscript).

81. Minutes, (n.79).

82. *Wis. Drugg.*, October, 1948, 8; ibid., February, 1949, 11; ibid., May, 1949, 8; ibid., July 1956, 14; ibid., June, 1957, 13; *Wis. Pharm.*, November, 1962, 346. In 1883, pharmacy students had been exempted from military drill. (Curti and Carstensen, (n. 5) I, 415)

83. *Wis. Drugg.*, December 1950, 7. In 1952, Kappa Epsilon was the largest professional society on the Madison campus. *Wis. Drugg.*, May, 1952, 8. In the mid–1950s, UWPhS was the only student branch in the nation to hold membership in the International Pharmaceutical Students' Federation. *Wis. Drugg.*, March, 1954, 15; ibid., March, 1955, 18.

84. *Wis. Drugg.*, November, 1951, 16; ibid., January, 1954, 10; ibid., January, 1955, 8; ibid., November, 1955, 11; ibid., December, 1957, 9; ibid., January, 1959, 10.

85. *Wis. Drugg.*, May, 1950, 27; ibid., June, 1956, 16; ibid., June, 1957, 12; ibid., October, 1957, 11. Zeta Chapter of Kappa Epsilon also hosted Grand Chapter meetings in 1927, 1937 and 1947. Marjorie M. Coghill, "The First Five Decades of Kappa Epsilon, 1921–1971," 1971, Kappa Epsilon Fraternity for Women Pharmacists, 43; *Wis. Drugg.*, May, 1947, 7. Region IV meetings of student branches of the APhA (SAPhA beginning in 1969) were also held in Madison in 1963 and 1977. *Wis. Pharm.*, March, 1963, 78; ibid., February, 1978, 64.

86. *Wis. Drugg.*, May, 1957, 9. Student Council was reorganized in the fall of 1964 with first occasional and then monthly meetings. In the 1960s, the Council concerned itself with student cheating, convocations, the High School Counseling Program of the School, organization of an All-Pharmacy Day and the institution of a common free hour during the day for meetings of organizations. *Mortar and Quill*, 4 (1966): No. 3, 17. During the 1970s the student Council became more prominent, with regular meetings and sponsorship of self-oriented activities.

87. *Wis. Drugg.*, October, 1945, 9; ibid., February, 1957, 11; *Wis. Pharm.*, February, 1967, 54. The class of 1980 published the only known yearbook, entitled "Showglobe," to have been exclusively devoted to pharmacy.

88. Originally, three issues of *Mortar and Quill* appeared during the school year. In 1966, a monthly newsletter was also published by the *Mortar and Quill* staff. The newsletter became bimonthly in 1970 and was published to the exclusion of larger *Mortar and Quill* issues. By 1974, *Mortar and Quill* reappeared and, since then, has published at a rate of two issues per school year.

89. *Mortar and Quill*, 4 (1965): No. 1, 4–5; *Mortar and Quill Newsletter*, 1B (1967): No. 6, 8; ibid., IB (1967): No. 8, 8 and 13; *Mortar and Quill*, Special Edition, "You and Your Environment," Spring, 1970; *Wis. Pharm.*, April, 1967, 143.

90. The purposes of Phi Delta Chi are "to advance the science of Pharmacy and its allied interests, and to foster and promote a fraternal spirit among its members." Originally, the object was "the advancement of pharmacy and chemistry" since its members were from both disciplines. But, by 1933, the objects were changed as the organization became composed exclusively of pharmacy students. Arndt, (n.52), 6–8; *The Badger Pharmacist*, (Madison, 1900), 141. In 1955, the pharmacy faculty ruled against reactivation of Phi Delta Chi since it "could result in no significant benefit at the present time, and, in fact, might actually jeopardize the activities of those organizations already established." (School of Pharmacy Faculty Minutes, January, 10, 1955, 3.)

91. The Madison Public Schools placed Delta chapter's Informational Slide Program on a recommended list of venereal disease references. (*Pill and Elixir*, (1973), No. 1)

92. When Phi Delta Chi modified its bylaws in 1976 to allow women members, Delta was the first among all chapters to comply. Also, it was the first among the pharmacy fraternities on the Madison campus to become coeducational. Kappa Psi began admitting women in the fall of 1977. In the spring of 1979, all of the Kappa Epsilon members were females and graduating seniors. The impending demise of the organization, in addition to the outmoded unisexual makeup of the group, stimulated the chapter to allow male members. The objects of the organization, however, remained the same. Conversations with James DeMuth and Perri Corrick-West, December 9, 1981; *Pill and Elixir*, 1976, Issue 19.

93. *Wis. Pharm.*, March, 1972, 72; ibid., September, 1977, 348; Scrapbook of Kappa Epsilon; conversation with Perri Corrick-West, December 9, 1981. The author appreciates the help of Jody Hein in the search for information about Kappa Epsilon.
94. *Wis. Pharm.*, April, 1973, 188; ibid., September, 1976, 307; *Mortar and Quill*, 4, (1966), No. 3, 19. The author thanks Virginia Lake for help in compiling information about Kappa Psi.
95. "Health Programs for the Community," Phi Delta Chi Professional Pharmacy Fraternity, (Madison, n.d.), 8 pp. Conversation with James DeMuth, December 9, 1981. Some of the information about Phi Delta Chi was kindly supplied by Mary Peterson.
96. *Wis. Pharm.*, May, 1967, 193; ibid., April, 1968, 134; ibid., April, 1969, 127; ibid., December, 1970, 465; ibid., November, 1972, 350; ibid., January, 1973, 19; ibid., April, 1976, 118; ibid., November, 1976, 372; ibid., July, 1978, 242; and personal experience of author. Between 1948 and 1970, UWPhS had an active branch at the Milwaukee Extension. This group held an annual spring banquet, set up window displays for Pharmacy Week and participated in Career Day. *Wis. Drugg.*, March, 1949, 7; ibid., June, 1950, 10; ibid., June, 1951, 29; ibid., July, 1955, 10; *Wis. Pharm.*, June, 1966, 249; conversation with Eunice Bardell, April 17, 1981.
97. The comprehensive examination was administered to senior students on the final day of University examinations as a means of ascertaining suitability for pharmacy practice. *Proc. WPhA, 1884*, 42. The award was described as follows: "The medal is of gold, the size of a twenty dollar gold piece; on one side the State coat of arms in raised and colored gold, on the reverse side, in enamel, the words 'Presented to for passing the best general examination at the School of Pharmacy, University of the State of Wisconsin', and around this, 'Wisconsin Pharmaceutical Association, 1885'." (*Proc. WPhA, 1885*, 25) Other recipients of the gold medal were Emil Weschcke, 1886; Charles A. Stilcke, 1887, Walter M. Carr, 1888 and Edward G. Raeuber, 1889. (KRF) In 1886, the Examining Committee gave special mention to Edward Kremers for his "great proficiency on the exam." (*Proc. WPhA, 1886*, 31) Also, in 1889, a special certificate was given to Alfred J. M. Lasche for "meritorious original investigation." (*Proc. WPhA, 1889*, 24) The desirability of awarding the gold medal was periodically debated until 1889 when, at the suggestion of students, it was discontinued on a motion from the Alumni Association. (*Proc. WPhA, 1889*, 16; *Wis. Drugg.*, April, 1940, 6). Power had probably made the original suggestion that a gold medal be awarded since he knew of such a prize given at Philadelphia College of Pharmacy commencement exercises. (E. Kremers, Report on Gold Medal, in KRF)
98. The list of names of the winners of the Rho Chi Award was compiled by Gregory J. Higby from the plaque in the School on which each name is engraved.
99. The list of names of the winners of the Eli Lilly Achievement Award was compiled by Gregory J. Higby from the plaque in the School on which each name is engraved.
100. Winners of the David Perlman Scholarship Award are permanently displayed on a plaque in the School of Pharmacy.
101. *Wis. Drugg.*, June, 1948, 9; *Wis. Pharm.*, August, 1967, 143; Coghill, (n.85), 45.

Research and Graduate Study

BY KENNETH A. CONNORS

RESEARCH in the School of Pharmacy began almost immediately after classes were initiated in 1883. Through the intervening century research activity has been continuous. Very shortly after the founding of the School, programs were offered leading to graduate degrees, the first Master of Science degree being awarded in 1893 and the first Doctor of Philosophy degree in 1902. The history of graduate study and research at the School of Pharmacy therefore must deal with the entire period of the School's existence. Chapter 5 surveys this history, and attempts also to evaluate the significance and impact of the research by faculty and students in the School of Pharmacy during the century 1883–1983.

Undergraduate Research

To the modern reader it is striking that the requirements for the Graduate in Pharmacy (Ph.G.) diploma (2-year course) included from the first year of instruction, 1883, a thesis based upon original research. The wording of this requirement in the initial college bulletin is not explicit:

> *". . . and shall submit an original essay or thesis upon some subject of Practical Pharmacy, Chemistry, Materia Medica, Botany, or other branch of science intimately connected therewith."*[1]

However, the interpretation given to the word "original" in this passage (presumably written by the Director, Frederick B. Power) usually included laboratory investigation. That Power should have initiated in Madison the first program in pharmacy in 1883 and expected the students from the first class (which graduated in 1885) to produce theses based upon original experimental work, and moreover that he succeeded in accomplishing this goal, tells us much about Power's capabilities and standards of excellence. Yet, ambitious as it was, this thesis requirement was not an innovative one at the time, for the best colleges of pharmacy had identical requirements. Thus the Philadelphia College of Pharmacy, from whose faculty Power had resigned to accept the Wisconsin position, required for the Ph.G. "an original dissertation, or thesis, upon some subject of Materia Medica, Pharmacy, Chemistry, or one of the branches of science immediately connected therewith . . ."[2]; the catalogs of the College of Pharmacy of the City of New York[3] and the Massachusetts College of Pharmacy[4] included similar requirements in 1883. Thus the Wisconsin curriculum, in this respect, was in the mainstream of contemporary pharmaceutical education.

We can learn something of Power's intentions and achievements by reading the theses that these pharmacy students submitted. Theses by the earliest classes have not survived, but there fortunately exists a formal research publication that summarizes the results. In 1885 the first published research from the Department of Pharmacy of the University of Wisconsin appeared as Number 1 in a series of contributions.[5] These articles were based on the student theses of the first graduating class. Their titles will give a sense of the topics of research interest at that time:

"The Medicinal Plants of the State of Wisconsin," Charles A. Foster.

"The Pharmacopoeial Application of Kerner's Test to Quinine and its Salts," F. B. Power and Henry G. Ruenzel.

"Examination of the Root of a Western Aconite," Frederick B. Power and Henry G. Ruenzel.

"Krameria Lanceolata Torrey," Henry F. Roberts.

"Determination of the Factors of Solubility of Some Officinal Chemicals," Frederick B. Power, with F. A. Scheuber, O. A. Kropf, and E. Naffz.

"Examination of Native Wines and Brandies," Oscar A. Kropf.

"The Insects Injurious to Drugs," Frithiof Kumlien.

"Analysis of a Solution of Bismuth and Hydrastine," Manford W. McMillen.

"The Crystalline Form and Solubility of Berberine and Some of Its Salts," William J. Huck.

"On the Constituents of the Rhizome of Hydrastis Canadensis Lin.," Frederick B. Power.

Some of the work reported in this publication was Power's personal research, and he was chiefly responsible also for guiding the students' research.

The contents of the second number of the *Contributions* commands attention especially because of the appearance in print of one of the class of 1886:[6]

> "A Yellow Opium Mold," Wm. Trelease.[7]
>
> "On Poppy Culture and Opium Production in the United States," Emil Weschcke.
>
> "Analysis of the Bark of Fraxinus Americana Lin. (White Ash)," Edward Kremers.
>
> "Examination of the Leaves of Aesculus Hippocastanum Lin. (Horse Chestnut)," Frederick O. Ray.
>
> "Examination of the So-Called Spruce-Gum," Adolph F. Menges.
>
> "Examination of the Leaves of Podophyllum Peltatum Lin.," Benjamin F. Carter.
>
> "Examination of the Root of Pastinaca Sativa Lin.," Joseph T. Bennett.
>
> "The Wild Parsnip (Pastinaca Sativa Lin.)," Frederick B. Power.
>
> "The Comparative Limits of Some Alkaloid Reactions and the Influence Exerted by Various Foreign Substances," Frank A. Rhyme.
>
> "On the Composition and Solubility of Strychnine Citrate," Frank H. Fischedick.

The name of special interest is, of course, Edward Kremers, who was to return (in 1890) as a member of the faculty, and who succeeded F. B. Power as Director of the Department.

The handwritten theses of the classes of 1887–92 have been preserved in collected bound volumes.[8] The handwriting is always legible, and in some instances is very handsome. Although some of the theses are little more than reviews ("term-papers" in later nomenclature), most of them include original laboratory work, some of it quite extensive. The level of scientific knowledge and sense of research purpose in some of these works is impressive, if it is recalled that they were developed and written during the second year of college training.

Beginning with the class of 1891, a sizeable fraction of the theses deal with chemical problems related to the terpenes. It was in 1890 that Edward Kremers joined the faculty, and he undoubtedly guided students to these problems, and directed the investigations for these theses (which, incidentally, tend to follow traditional models of scientific writing more closely than do others not obviously stimulated by Kremers, for example by copious citation of the literature). Many theses of this period cite papers by Kremers in their bibliographies. In 1891 W. C. Wallschlaeger's thesis dealt with the components of the bark of the white ash, clearly following up Kremers' own Ph.G. thesis work as published in the *Contributions*.[6]

By 1897, theses were being typed and individually bound.[9] Examples exist of both Ph.G. and B.Sc. (Pharmacy) theses.[8] Most of them reported laboratory investigations, but some were reviews or bibliographies. The B.Sc. thesis of Irvin W. Brandel (1901) was titled "Bibliography of Volatile Oils"; it ran to 537 pages, plus an author index. This work must have been of great value to Professor Kremers in his own research studies. In 1900 a *joint* Ph.G. thesis of 125 pages, titled "On Oils Containing Cineol and Phellandrene," was submitted by Albert N. Tandvig and Harry Klueter; this included an extensive bibliography and experimental results. It is worth mentioning the 1897 B.Sc. thesis ("A Study of Aqueous Soap Solutions") of Oswald Schreiner, who a few years later was awarded the first Ph.D. degree in pharmaceutical studies. The 1911 Ph.G. thesis of Oscar Rennebohm, later a prominent Madison pharmacist, regent of the University, and governor of the state of Wisconsin, was a literature review and systematization titled "Periodic Literature on New Remedies."

The description of the thesis requirement, as modified in the 1893–1894 *Bulletin*, gives some notion of the scheduling and effort that was expected:

> *"The student may select the subject of his thesis from either botany or chemistry, general or applied, provided he be found proficient by the instructor under whose personal supervision he chooses to carry out such work. About a term and a half, four hours daily, are expected to be given to the necessary laboratory experiments. However, time is not the only criterion."*[10]

The thesis research was a major component of the undergraduate program until shortly after World War II.[11] This change was a consequence of the large enrollment increase and the corresponding difficulty in supervising substantial research projects for all students. Occasional Bachelor's theses continued to be presented, however, and the course titled Thesis (now numbered 691, 692) is still available to undergraduate students, and is still elected by a small number of them.

Despite the reduction in undergraduate research activity resulting from the removal of a thesis as a degree requirement, a very active program of research by undergraduate students exists at the present time. The vehicle is course number 699, Advanced Independent Study, through which qualified students may carry out original research under the direction of a faculty member. In the period 1967–81, 16.4% of pharmacy students registered in this course, and much of the research conducted by these students led to publications in the technical and scholarly literature.

Graduate Degree Programs

Program Development. As we have seen, F. B. Power initiated research work at the School and established research as an activity appropriate to pharmaceutical training. But Power left the University in 1892, and his successor as Director, Edward Kremers, was responsible for the development of programs leading to graduate degrees, and for the idea that the training of pharmaceutical scientists, as well as of pharmacy practitioners, is a proper function of the School of Pharmacy.

It was clearly not possible to offer a graduate degree until a baccalaureate program was in place, and the (optional) 4-year Bachelor of Science program was first offered in 1892.[12] The Master of Pharmacy degree, which could be taken by graduates of the 2-year (or later 3-year) program upon completion of a further year of advanced study, had been offered for the first time in 1891–92; but this cannot be considered a graduate degree in a strict academic sense because the baccalaureate was not a prerequisite. Nevertheless, the Ph.M. program clearly was a model for a formal graduate program. The nature and the timing of its introduction seem characteristic of Kremers' eagerness for innovation and his ability to adapt to

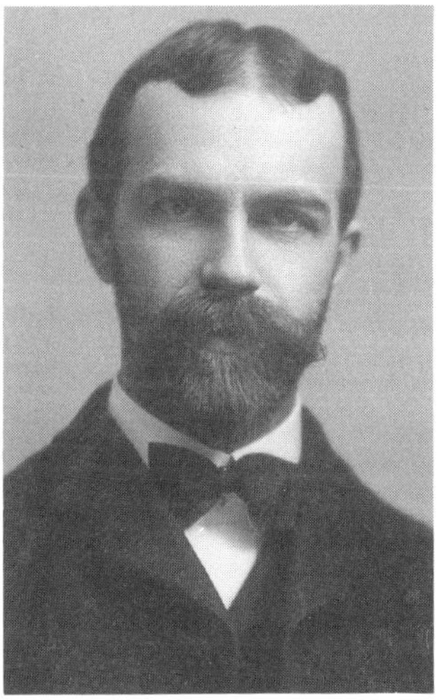

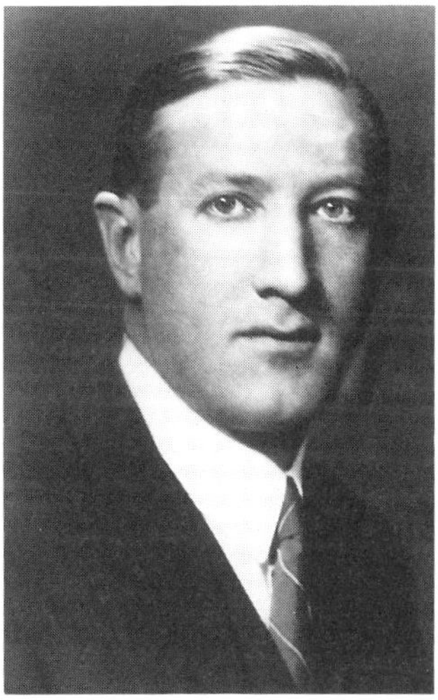

The first pharmacy graduate to attain a Ph.D. in the USA under supervision of a member of a pharmacy faculty was the chemist Oswald Schreiner (left), who made a life-long career in the U.S. Department of Agriculture. The School had been authorized to provide Ph.D. programs independently by 1917 when a Ph.D. (pharmaceutics) was conferred on the Wisconsin pharmacist Andrew G. DuMez (right), whose prominent career included the deanship at the University of Maryland.

administrative requirements. Only three Ph.M. degrees were awarded (in 1894, 1902, and 1907).

The Master of Science degree program was first offered in the 1894–95 *Bulletin*. It is further evidence of Kremers' drive in developing the School, that the first M.S. in Pharmacy was awarded (to John L. Mead) in 1893! This was possible because Mead (who had earned a UW Ph.G. degree) held a non-pharmacy Bachelor's degree (Lawrence, 1888).[13] The first M.S. in Pharmacy based on a Wisconsin B.Sc. in Pharmacy was awarded to Oswald Schreiner in 1899.[14]

The first Doctor of Philosophy degree supervised from this School was awarded to Oswald Schreiner in 1902. This statement requires amplification. Stieb has closely examined the circumstances.[13] At the time, the School of Pharmacy was not empowered to offer a Ph.D. program in Pharmacy, and Schreiner's degree was in Chemistry, with the thesis research directed by Kremers, the Professor of Pharmacy. The distinction, of which Kremers was well aware, was between a degree awarded for work in a pharmaceutical department (which Schreiner's was) and a degree with a major in Pharmacy (which was not, at the time, administratively possible).[15] The first Ph.D. from this School with a major in Pharmacy was awarded in 1917 to Andrew G. DuMez, whose thesis was titled "The Oleoresins of the United States Pharmacopoeia." In current terminology, Schreiner in 1902 received the first Ph.D. in Pharmaceutical Chemistry, and DuMez in 1917 took the first Ph.D. in Pharmaceutics.

Although European science education was an example to Kremers, his boldness as an innovator in American pharmaceutical education was remarkable. The University had admitted the study of Pharmacy in 1883, but it was not widely regarded as an academic discipline. Within 10 years Kremers had produced the B.Sc., M.S., and Ph.D. programs, and had trained the first Ph.D. candidate. This is especially notable when one learns that the first Ph.D. degree in any field at the University of Wisconsin was granted in 1892.

These pharmaceutical Ph.D. programs were the first of their kind in the United States. In later decades similar enterprise was shown by the faculty in developing graduate degree programs in other specialty areas. The first Ph.D. in the History of Pharmacy, in America, was awarded in 1952 to Glenn A. Sonnedecker; historical studies had been one of Kremers' interests, and the School's capabilities in this field had been greatly strengthened with the addition to the faculty of Professor George Urdang in 1947. The Ph.D. in Pharmacy Administration, one of the earliest in America, though not the first, was first awarded in 1954 to William S.

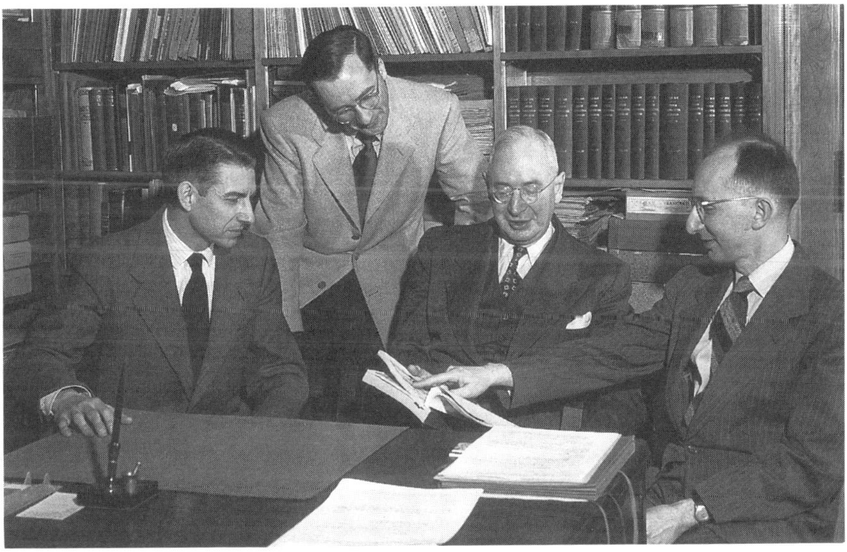

The UW reputation as a national center for cultivating the history of pharmacy was much enhanced, internationally, with the appointment of Professor George Urdang as the first full-time historian. He is shown (holding book) with three graduate students about 1950: (l. to r.) Glenn Sonnedecker, Garnet R. Paterson, and Alex Berman.

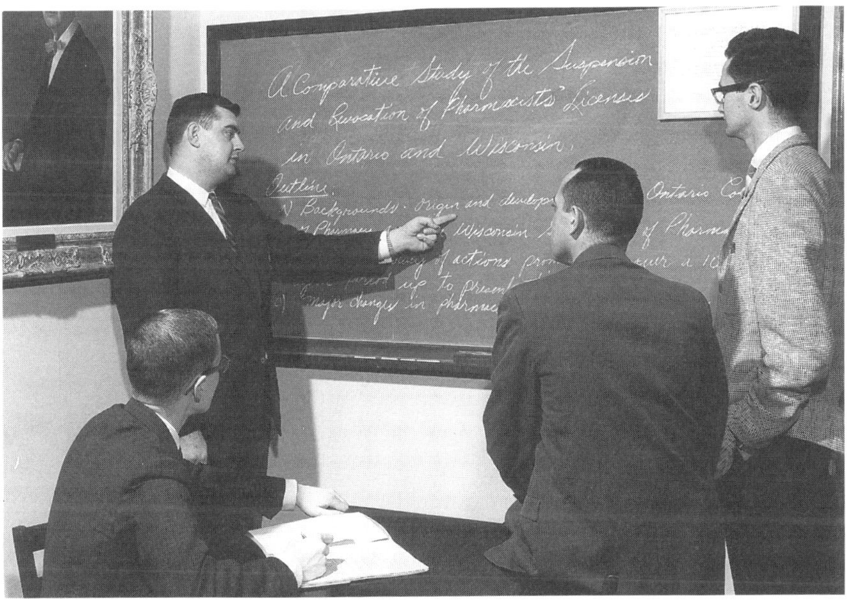
A Comparative Study of the Suspension
and Revocation of Pharmacists' Licenses
in Ontario and Wisconsin.
Outline

Social studies of contemporary pharmacy at UW was the first such graduate program in the USA. The first four graduate students are shown discussing a project in 1965. Sociologist Bonnie L. Svarstad took charge of the program in 1975, the first full-time professor.

Apple. In 1963 the first American graduate program devoted to the Social Studies of Pharmacy was initiated at this School, and in 1966 the first such program in Pharmaceutical Extension instruction was begun.

The Graduate Students. Graduate studies in the School of Pharmacy can be seen, from our present viewpoint, to have been divided into two general periods: there was the formative-traditional period, ranging from 1893 through the end of World War II; and the modern period, starting about 1950. This division is clearly revealed in Figures 5.1 and 5.2 (below), showing numbers of graduate degrees awarded by year. For both Master's and Doctor of Philosophy degrees the same pattern is seen, with small numbers of graduates in the early years, a rise beginning in the late 1920s, a drop during the depression and the war years, then the substantial postwar increase.[16] Some of the scatter in Figure 5.1 probably results from the policy that the Master's degree is not a requirement for the Ph.D.; whether the M.S. is taken depends in part upon the field of study, the contemporary philosophy of the faculty in that field, and the student's wishes. During the first century, 483 Master's degrees and 414 Ph.D. degrees were earned in the School of Pharmacy (see *Appendix 4d*, p. 209).

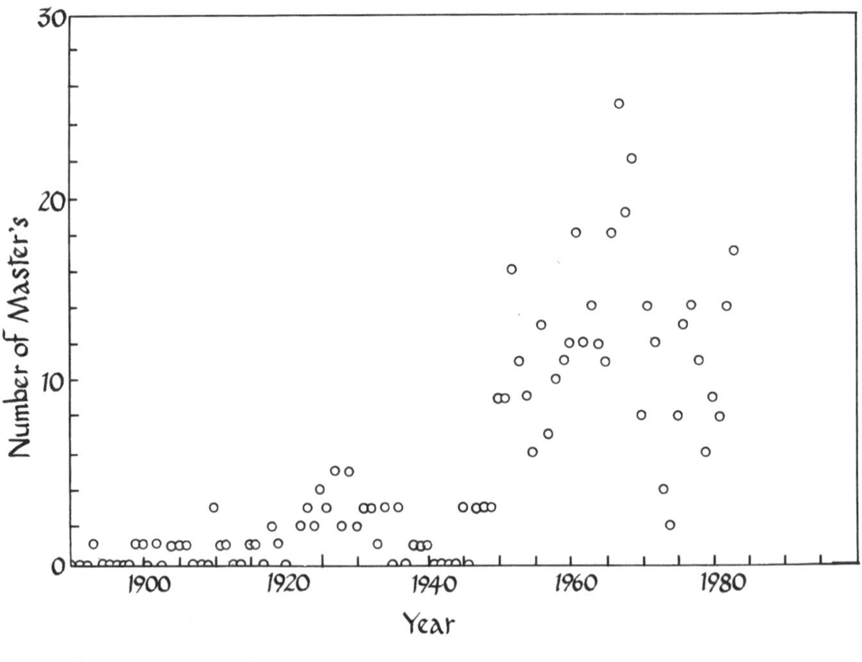

Figure 5.1. Master's degrees awarded, by year, for graduate work in the School of Pharmacy.

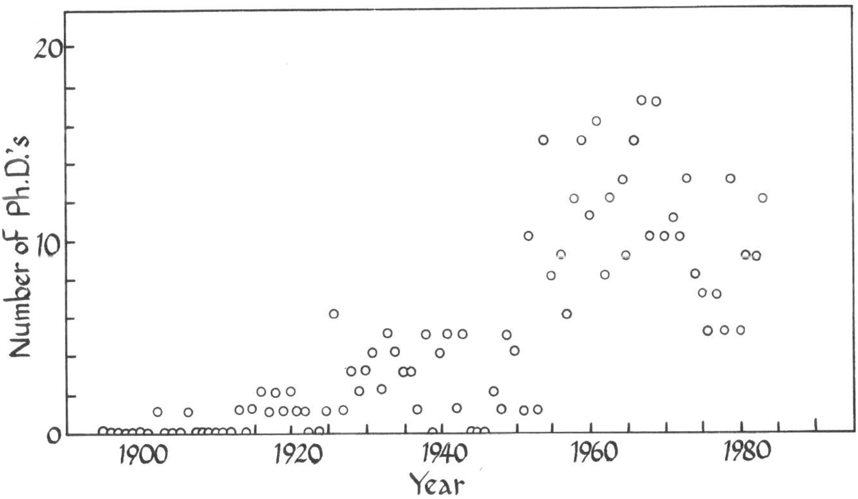

Figure 5.2. Doctor of Philosophy degrees awarded, by year, for work in School of Pharmacy.

Just as the numbers of degrees increased sharply after 1950, so too did the number of graduate faculty, as described in the following section. In consequence, the nature of the research embodied in Master's and Ph.D. theses is markedly different in the traditional and modern (post–1950) periods. Before World War II much thesis research could be described as plant chemistry, pharmacognosy, or medicinal organic chemistry. During the modern period a wider range of research topics is reflected in thesis titles, with a majority being in physical pharmacy and pharmaceutics; during this period, also, are seen titles in pharmacy administration, historical studies and other social studies of pharmacy, and, beginning in the 1960s, in pharmacology. Among Master's thesis titles hospital pharmacy (administrative and clinical) contribute largely in the 1970s. The M.B.A. degrees awarded in the period 1951–62 were for theses in pharmacy administration; subsequent Master's candidates in this field were awarded the M.S.

The total numbers of graduate students in the School have fluctuated widely. The table (*Appendix 4b*, p. 204) lists the graduate student enrollment from 1950 on; during this period the population ranged between 46 and 95 students. Several factors have influenced graduate student enrollment, including the number of faculty and their research fields and reputations, availability of graduate student stipends (through fellowships, teaching assistantships, and research assistantships), recruitment efforts, alternative career opportunities, and competing graduate programs in other schools of pharmacy. This last factor probably played a role in defining the patterns seen in Figures 5.1 and 5.2, for in the 1950s Wisconsin was pre-eminent in several graduate areas, most notably in physical pharmacy; later, as other schools of pharmacy developed strong graduate programs, the Wisconsin enrollment and numbers of degrees awarded ceased to exhibit the remarkable rate of increase seen early in the modern period.

What proportion of the graduate students were earlier undergraduates at Wisconsin? Historical data yield interesting answers (with respect to B.Sc. degrees in two periods)[17]: We find, for the years 1893–1934, that 26 of 54 Master's degrees (48%) and 17 of 48 Ph.D. degrees (35%) were awarded to holders of the UW B.Sc. in Pharmacy. For the period 1954–64, 21 of 124 Master's degrees (17%) and 18 of 125 Ph.D. degrees (14%) were taken by UW B.Sc. (Pharmacy) graduates. The data for the earlier period reveal that from the first years of the graduate program it attracted students from outside the School of Pharmacy, often from other UW departments. In the post-World War II era, many of these students came from other American schools of pharmacy, as well as from overseas institutions.[18]

The first woman to earn the Master's degree was Florence Meta Gage (M.S., 1900), who had taken the B.Sc. in 1898. Nellie A. Wakeman was the first woman to be awarded the Ph.D. (in 1913); Dr. Wakeman, who also held the B.Sc. (1908) and M.S. (1910) in pharmacy from UW, served on the faculty of the School from 1913 to 1946. Significant numbers of women have earned graduate degrees in the modern period, but the percentages remain small: over the century, 70 of 483 Master's degrees (14.5%) and 30 of 414 Ph.D. degrees (7.2%).[19]

The percentage of pharmacy baccalaureate graduates who choose to pursue advanced studies for a graduate degree will probably always be small, because the choice of a professional program at the undergraduate level is a career decision unlikely to lead to the necessary motivation for research training. Nevertheless, modest numbers of undergraduate pharmacy students have, throughout the century, altered their career goals and elected to pursue graduate study. The class of 1965 is a remarkable example; of this class of 72 B.Sc. graduates, at least 10 earned M.S. degrees and 12 earned Ph.D. degrees (10 of the doctorates being taken at this School).

The Graduate Faculty. The graduate faculty of the University is comprised of those faculty who are entitled, by the rules of the University, to supervise graduate students in the sense of acting as thesis advisers ("major professors"). These are faculty holding the positions of Assistant

Professor, Associate Professor, or Professor. Figure 5.3 (below) is a plot of the number of graduate faculty members in the School of Pharmacy by year.[20] This plot is a sigmoid growth curve, the greatest rate of change occurring in the two decades 1950 to 1970. At the end of the first century the size of the graduate faculty appears to have stabilized at about 30 members. (The total faculty size continues to grow, the increase being in the clinical faculty.)

The composition of the faculty, in the sense of the areas of research, has altered as it has grown. Some of the directions of this development have been mentioned above. Throughout the traditional period the research strengths were in pharmacognosy and medicinal chemistry, with some interest in galenical pharmacy. In the 1940s there began a qualitative change in the make-up of the faculty with the addition of several members whose research interests were physical-chemical rather than classically medicinal-chemical. This movement was initiated and stimulated by Louis W. Busse and Joseph V. Swintosky, and in the 1950s its primary leaders were Dale E. Wurster and, especially, Takeru Higuchi, who had been trained as a physical chemist in the UW chemistry department. The field

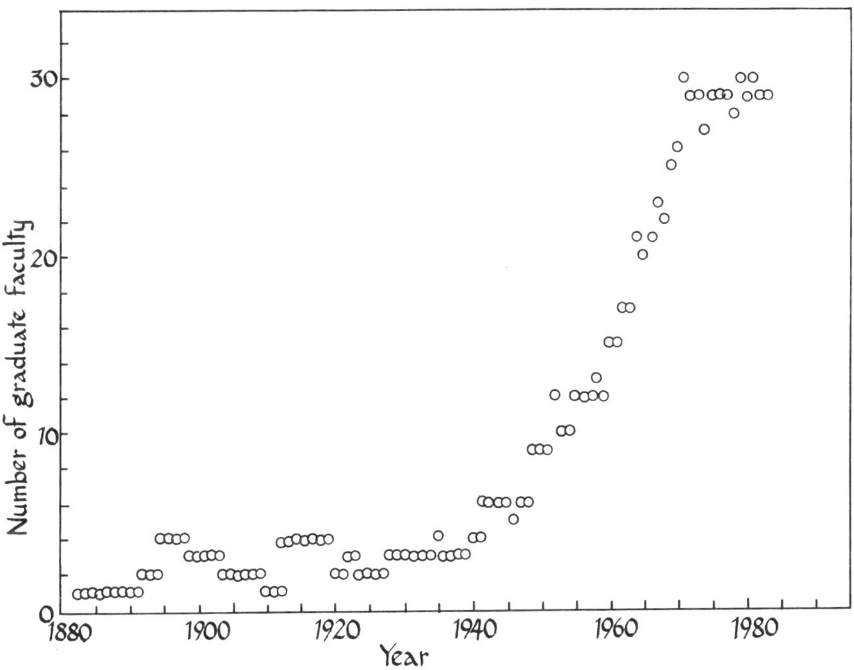

Figure 5.3. Number of graduate faculty in the School of Pharmacy by year.

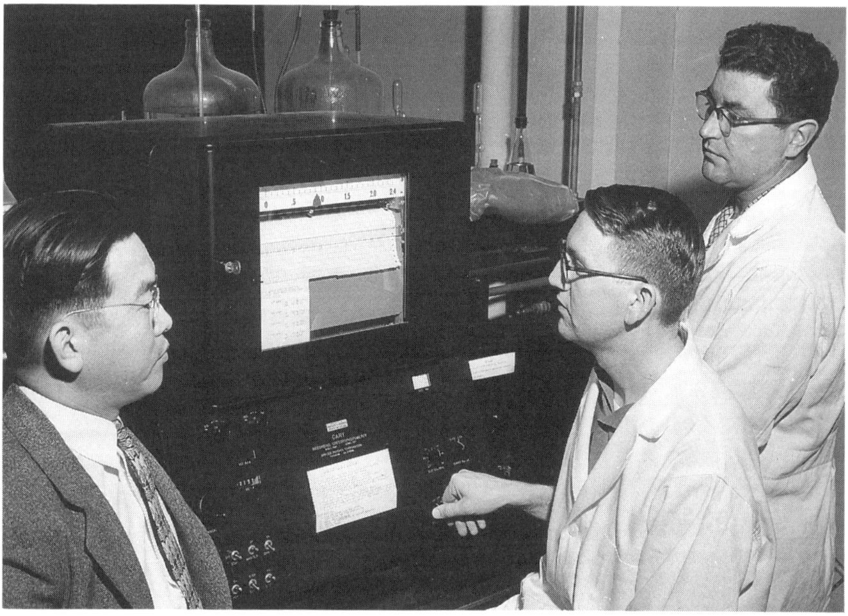

By applying physical chemistry to pharmaceutical problems, beginning in the 1940s, Professor Takeru Higuchi (left) and associates gave a new direction nationally to pharmaceutics research.

developed by these Wisconsin researchers became known as physical pharmacy (the application of physical-chemical methods to pharmaceutical problems). In later years, broadened by the addition of studies of biological systems, it developed into the field currently called pharmaceutics, or the study of drug delivery systems in all their aspects. During the three decades of this modern period the graduate faculty group in pharmaceutics has undergone considerable growth and change in membership; since about 1960 it has included eight faculty members.

The medicinal chemistry area was dominated during the rapid growth phase of the faculty (see Figure 5.3) by S. Morris Kupchan, who continued and extended the tradition of sound research in organic medicinals and biologically active materials from natural sources. The medicinal chemistry group has, throughout the modern period, consisted of 3 or 4 graduate-faculty members. During this period another group of researchers, denoted the pharmaceutical biochemistry group, and led during the growth phase by Charles J. Sih and David Perlman, explored biochemical mechanisms and microbial transformations, with some areas of interest in common with the medicinal chemists.

Pharmacological research and graduate training is a relatively recent addition to the School's programs, beginning with the addition of

Kenneth F. Finger to the faculty in 1962. This faculty group grew to six members by 1980.

The School has long been noted for its historical research. Edward Kremers, though not a professional historian, had a strong interest in the history of pharmacy. Since 1947, when George Urdang joined the faculty after a distinguished career in Germany, the history of pharmacy has been one of the areas of graduate study at this School. Glenn Sonnedecker led this program for over three decades, and collaborated closely with the UW Department of the History of Science. Associated with this area, and

TABLE 5.1. Graduate Faculty Who Served 10 Years or More[a] During the First Century.

Name	*Years Served*	*Name*	*Years Served*
F.B. Power	10	J.R. Arndt	17
J.J. Windheuser	10	P. Mukerjee	17
E.W. Stieb	10	J.R. Robinson	18
H.A. Langenhan	11	A.P. Lemberger	19
L.S. Cheney	12	P.A. Hart	20
J.H. Perrin	12	W.L. Blockstein	20
G. Zografi	12	L.M. Parks	20
P.G. Welling	12	T. Higuchi	21
S.M. Kupchan	13	E.B. Bardell	21
T.A. Rudy	13	K.A. Connors	22
G.L. Amidon	13	D.E. Wurster	24
D.B. Northrop	13	C.J. Sih	24
D.H. Rich	14	R.W. Hammel	25
D. Perlman	14	W.O. Richtmann	31
P. Bass	14	G. Sonnedecker	31
C.K. Buckner	14	N.A. Wakeman	34
J.L. Parascandola	14	A.H. Uhl	38
M.H. Weinswig	15	L.W. Busse	39
R. Fischer	16	E. Kremers	45
J.T. Carstensen	16		

[a]Compiled from list of faculty (Appendix 2); years served include service as Instructor, Assistant Professor, Associate Professor, and Professor between 1883 and 1983.

housed in the School, is the American Institute of the History of Pharmacy, which was founded here in 1941. Research in pharmacy administration began with William S. Apple, who joined the faculty in 1954. Continuing education graduate study developed from the program in extension services, which was initiated by Louis W. Busse.[21]

For a faculty member to have a significant impact on graduate education and research direction within the School, an effort continuing over a period of at least several years is necessary. Although it is not possible to establish the minimum number of years required to have a major influence, it involves a commitment to the School that comprises a significant portion of the scholar's professional career. Therefore, Table 5.1 lists those members of the graduate faculty who have served the School of Pharmacy for 10 years or more during the century 1883–1983.

Research Activities and Accomplishments

The Pharmaceutical Experiment Station.[22] In the two-decade period 1913 to 1933 a remarkable research organization developed and flourished at the School of Pharmacy in Madison. The organization, or arrangement, was called the Wisconsin Pharmaceutical Experiment Station; it was patterned after state agriculture stations, but it was the first such venture in the pharmaceutical field in the United States. Edward Kremers was its director and driving force.

Although the statutory origin of the Pharmaceutical Experiment Station may be placed at 1913, the development stage went back to 1895, when Dr. Rodney H. True was appointed Assistant Professor of pharmacognosy. True left Wisconsin in 1899, lectured briefly at Harvard University, and then in 1901 took a position in a newly created Office of Drug-Plant and Poisonous-Plant Investigations in the Bureau of Plant Industry of the U.S. Department of Agriculture in Washington, D.C. True and Kremers shared scientific interests, and ultimately the relationship led to an institutional cooperation. In the spring and summer of 1908 Kremers, with the help of pharmacy students and his children, grew a small drug garden on his own property. True, visiting Madison, was sufficiently impressed that he transferred the northern station of his office from Vermont to Wisconsin, and he proposed a cooperative experiment between the USDA Office of Drug-Plant and Poisonous-Plant Investigations and the UW Department of Pharmacy.

In 1909 this cooperative project was undertaken on a two and one-half acre site in Camp Randall, chosen, it was said, "not because it afforded

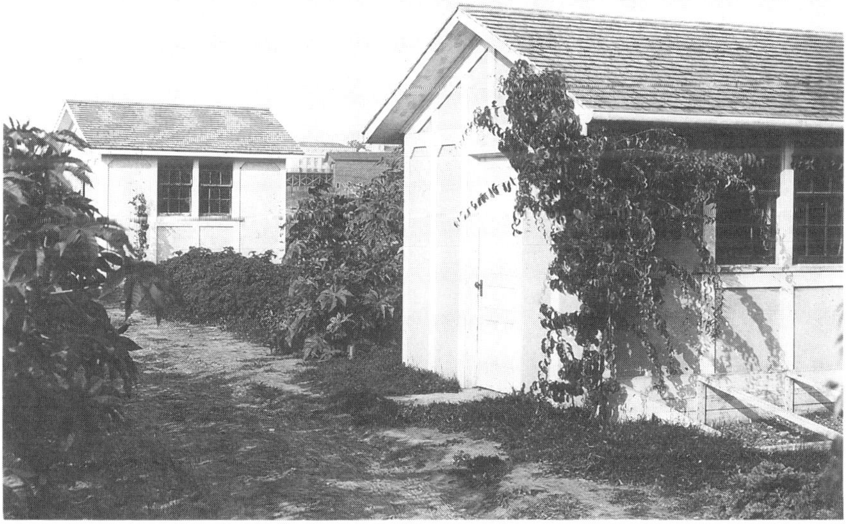

The Pharmaceutical Experiment Station (f. 1913) ranged from the growing of medicinal plants experimentally to the characterizing of chemical constituents. At the entrance to the School's acreage (above) were cold frames, a drying shed, and tool shed. Below, graduate students are shown experimenting with the botanical drugs harvested.

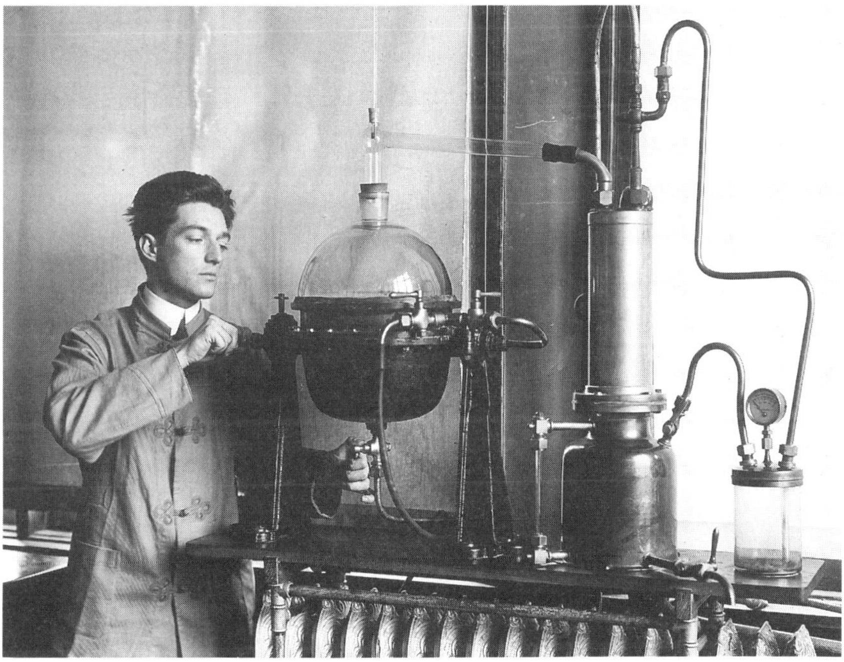

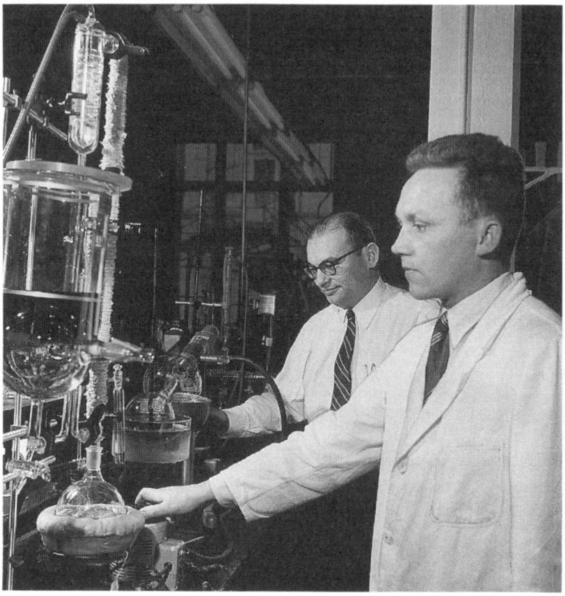

Graduate-student laboratories, such as this one in medicinal chemistry, have been an essential part of the School since the turn of the century. During the 1950s Professor Morris Kupchan (left) was involving these students in research on alkaloids, sterols, and growth factors.

good soil but because it was agreed upon by all that this was the one spot on the campus where the garden would be least likely of disturbance."[22] In 1910 the Bureau of Plant Industry requested addition of another acre to the garden. A fence, tool shed, cold frame, drying shed, and still house were constructed. According to the official agreement of 1909, the University was responsible for supplying the land, the cultivation, and related needs, whereas the USDA Bureau of Plant Industry was to supply seeds and plants, as well as an expert, who spent spring, summer, and fall in Madison, and the winter in Washington. A later "Memorandum of Understanding between the University of Wisconsin, Course of Pharmacy, and the Bureau of Plant Industry of the U.S. Dept. of Agriculture" (1912) stipulated that the University furnish a piece of land not to exceed three acres, the necessary labor and horses, and the fertilizer, the value not to exceed $150 annually; the use of the pharmacy laboratory was also given. The Bureau was to furnish additional help and apparatus, to a limit of $150. The Bureau also reserved the right to publish results obtained from both the garden and the laboratory.

This "cooperative experiment" resulted in the production of high-quality drug plants in sufficient quantity for extensive laboratory investigation. At the time, of course, most of the potent drugs available for therapy were of plant origin, and the materials commercially available to pharmacists and physicians could be of uncertain purity and strength.[23] The drug garden was a source of reliable plant materials for systematic laboratory investigations on the production, analysis, chemical properties, and pharmaceutical formulation of drugs. In addition, the garden was an experiment in the possibility of the commercial production of plant drugs. In fact, at this stage of the development of the cooperative experiment, it was agreed that the portion of the crop of 1913 that was in excess of that needed for laboratory investigations be placed at the disposal of the pharmacists of the state of Wisconsin.

At the annual meeting of the Wisconsin Pharmaceutical Association in June of 1912, in Delavan, a resolution was unanimously voted to the effect that its legislative committee seek passage of a bill for the establishment of the first pharmaceutical station in the United States. Bill No. 247S was enacted the following year and was signed by Governor Francis E. McGovern on June 2, 1913. In this way the cooperative experiment between the "Course in Pharmacy" and the USDA became a statutory unit, the Wisconsin Pharmaceutical Experiment Station, the first such unit in the country. In the 1913–14 UW Bulletin of the Department of Pharmacy the law is quoted, and because it clearly outlines the goals of the Station it is repeated here:

> CHAPTER 404, LAWS OF 1913
>
> AN ACT to create section 392em–12, and subsection 21 of section 172–53 of the statutes, relating to a pharmaceutical experiment station at the state university, and making an appropriation.
>
> The people of the state of Wisconsin, represented in Senate and Assembly, do enact as follows:
>
> Section 1. There is added to the statutes a new section and, to section 172–53, a new subsection of the statutes, to read: Section 392em–12. The board of regents of the state university are authorized and directed to establish, equip and maintain in the department of pharmacy of the state university a pharmaceutical experiment station. The duties of the said station shall be
>
> (1) To cooperate with the bureau of plant industry of the department of agriculture in the maintenance of the northern station for the cultivation of medicinal plants and to disseminate such information as may lead to the proper cultivation of medicinal plants and the production of high grade vegetable drugs in this state; and

(2) To serve the public at large by cooperation with both pharmacists and physicians in securing for the sick the best medicines that pharmaceutical science and art can provide, and further by cooperation with the state board of pharmacy, the state board of health, and the dairy and food commission to bring about these results.

(Section 172–53.) 2. There is annually appropriated on July 1 twenty-five hundred dollars, payable from any moneys in the general fund, not otherwise appropriated, to the regents of the university for the department of pharmacy, to carry out the provisions of section 392em–12.

Section 2. This act shall take effect upon passage and publication.

Approved June 2, 1913.

For the next 20 years the Pharmaceutical Experiment Station served as the research branch of the Department of Pharmacy. Edward Kremers was the director for the whole of this period, and the staff, besides Kremers, consisted generally of a pharmacognosist, a chemist, a gardener, a secretary, and a variable number of research assistants, who were graduate students in the department.[24] Some of the staff were evidently jointly appointed with the station and the Department, as indicated by this 1917–18 proposed budget:[25]

Director, Edward Kremers	
Chemist, Emerson R. Miller	$ 800
Pharmacist, Henry A. Langenhan	100
Pharmacognosist, Rollin H. Denniston	100
Stenographer, Irene Dengel	480
Gardener, George Bents	600
Horse,	100
Equipment and supplies,	320
	$2500

In 1917 two factors brought about the displacement of the drug garden from Camp Randall. One of these was the increased acreage required to accommodate the activities of the growing Pharmaceutical Experiment Station; the other was the need to yield to "athletic interests." The Board of Regents assigned a 40-acre site (known as the "Olin Forty") to the Pharmaceutical Experiment Station. By 1918 ten acres were under cultivation. The Olin Forty site was near Picnic Point, about two and one-half miles northwest of the Department of Pharmacy.[26]

As the first organization of its kind, the Pharmaceutical Experiment Station attracted considerable attention throughout the country and the world.[22] Professional and technical journals commented favorably upon its goals and achievements, and called for its emulation in other states. The times, however, were working against the Experiment Station, and the great depression ended it when the Wisconsin legislature terminated the annual appropriation in 1933. Cultivation of the pharmaceutical garden continued for several years, but Edward Kremers' retirement in 1935 brought to a close this innovative experience in pharmaceutical research and service.

[In the 1990s new problems and opportunities led to the resurrection of the idea of the Pharmaceutical Experiment Station (which continued to be authorized by statute) as a drug development service to provide research and development capabilities to University inventors and discoverers of substances having potential pharmaceutical applications. The purpose of this modern version of the Station is to furnish preformulation, formulation, and manufacture of clinical supplies, taking a drug from its discovery stage to the clinical testing stage. Licensing to commercial interests may ultimately lead to financial benefits to the School of Pharmacy and the University.]

Research Facilities. The physical location of the School of Pharmacy has been treated in other chapters, and it is sufficient here to outline some of the facilities for research and scholarly studies that have been available to faculty and students. The drug garden was a major research facility from 1909 to the late 1930s, as described in the preceding section on the Wisconsin Pharmaceutical Experiment Station.

In the early years, when the School was housed in South Hall and then in North Hall, evidently research was carried out in the same laboratories that were used for undergraduate instruction, although Power had a private laboratory after 1884. As soon as the "new" Chemistry Building was completed (in 1905), the School moved to it from North Hall, and from that time increases in space for research and instruction have been achieved by successive administrations of the School.

From time to time remodelling of laboratories has been carried out to bring them to contemporary standards for research work. At the end of its first century, the School of Pharmacy occupied all of the West and East wings of Chamberlin Hall, but laboratory research and library facilities were left without room for expansion of programs.[27] An important shift in the character of research from chemical investigations to studies using living systems (including microorganisms, cells, mammals, birds, and fish) has put additional strains on research facilities designed as chemical laboratories. Even after relocation of the library and the animal-care facility

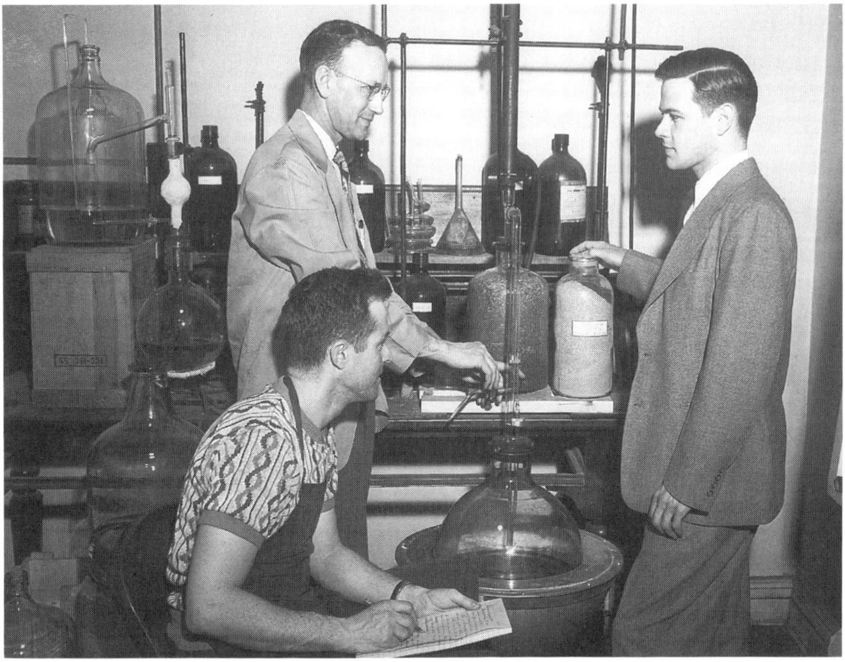

Research degrees in medicinal chemistry have been one major focus of the School's graduate program since its beginning. A graduate student's problem is discussed (above, standing l. to r.) by Professors Lloyd M. Parks and William Foye, in the 1950s. One of their successors, Professor Daniel Rich is shown (below) preparing an experiment, about 1971.

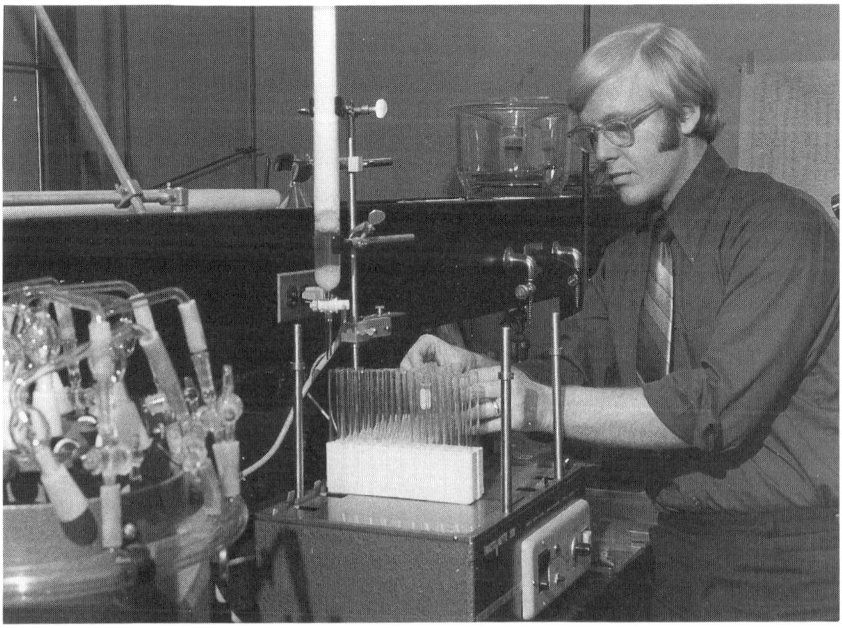

(1988–89), it was clear that obtaining a modern building designed for pharmaceutical education (as many other schools of pharmacy had achieved) would have to receive priority.

Conferences and Lectures. One of the ways in which the research environment is enriched and researchers are stimulated is by personal interaction with outstanding contemporary researchers. Besides the School of Pharmacy seminar program that has offered each curricular area periodic opportunities to invite speakers to the School, some annual named lectureships have been instituted to bring distinguished researchers to the Madison campus to describe their work. The Rennebohm Lectures of the School of Pharmacy, supported by the Oscar Rennebohm Foundation, date from 1955. The Rennebohm Lecturers, and their topics, are listed in *Appendix 7* (p. 223). Besides providing students and faculty with exposure to leading researchers and issues, this lecture series has constituted a notable contribution to UW campus culture.

Upon the retirement of Professor Louis W. Busse from the faculty in 1978, the Louis W. Busse Pharmacy Lectures were instituted as an annual lectureship designed to bring outstanding lecturers on industrial pharmaceutical topics to the campus. The L. W. Busse Lecturers and their subjects are given in *Appendix 8* (p. 227).

The School faculty, through the University, has also honored some of its graduates and former associates by awarding them UW honorary degrees or citations for distinguished service to pharmacy. Many of those awarded have made their careers in research. The list of recipients is given in *Appendix 5* (p. 215).

The School of Pharmacy has served as a focus or unifying influence on research trends by acting as a sponsor of conferences or symposia. An important event of this type was the Seventh Meeting of the American Peptide Symposium, which was organized by Daniel H. Rich of the School of Pharmacy; 550 participants from 20 countries participated in this 1981 conference.[28]

Late in the 1950s the idea was conceived, principally by Louis W. Busse and Takeru Higuchi, of having a small pharmaceutical research conference to deal mainly with scientific problems of pharmaceutical formulation, production, and performance. Here industrial and academic scientists could exchange ideas in both formal (lecture) and informal settings. The first of these conferences (formally titled the National Industrial Pharmaceutical Research Conferences) was held in 1959, and meetings have been held annually since. Table 5.2 (p. 153) gives the conference subjects and attendance. For about 15 years these conferences were held in the

King's Gateway Hotel in Land O' Lakes, Wisconsin, 250 miles north of Madison on the Wisconsin-Michigan border, consequently they became informally but widely known as the "Land O' Lakes Conferences." In the late 1970s the Land O' Lakes site became unavailable, and the conference was moved to Lake Delton, Wisconsin, and still later to Devil's Head Resort, but it is still referred to as the Land O' Lakes Conference. The typical meeting format consists of lecture presentations in the morning and evening, with afternoons free for informal discussions and recreation. The informal nature, relatively isolated setting, and limited attendance of the Land O' Lakes Conferences have worked together to generate highly stimulating, productive, and enjoyable meetings for pharmaceutical scientists.

With the success of the Land O' Lakes Conferences devoted to problems in pharmaceutics (usually held in June), it became clear that a similar need existed in pharmaceutical analysis, and the annual Land O' Lakes Conferences on Pharmaceutical Analysis were inaugurated in 1961. These analytical conferences have usually been organized around techniques and problems, and eventually have included optional afternoon "workshops" and problem-solving sessions. The Land O' Lakes Conferences have been sponsored and produced jointly by the School of Pharmacy and Extension Services in Pharmacy.

In 1996 the first Madison Conference on the Pharmaceutical Sciences was presented. This activity of the Division of Pharmaceutical Sciences is planned as a biennial meeting of faculty, graduate students, and research alumni.

Scholarly Activities of the Faculty. Research is disseminated primarily in technical journals; and the hundreds of publications by the School's faculty have fulfilled the creative function that is part of the obligation of any university faculty. The nature of such pharmaceutical research at Wisconsin is described in the next section. The present section takes note of other kinds of scholarly work and its recognition.

Faculty members of this School have been widely recognized by election to office in professional associations, including the American Pharmaceutical Association (APhA), the Academy of Pharmaceutical Sciences (APS), the American Association for the Advancement of Science (AAAS), the American Chemical Society (ACS), the American Association of Pharmaceutical Scientists (AAPS), the International Academy of the History of Pharmacy, and others. Such offices represent a service by the office-holder to the profession, and are not in themselves a form of scholarly work; but they are a form of recognition for contributions to the field. For example, four members of the faculty (L. W. Busse, T. Higuchi, A. P.

TABLE 5.2. The National Industrial Pharmaceutical Research Conferences (Land O' Lakes Conferences)

Year	*Topic*	*Attendance*
1959	Pharmaceutical Aspects of Tabletting	131
1960	Stability and Stabilization of Pharmaceuticals	179
1961	Physical Stability of Dispersed Systems	151
1962	Pharmaceutical Solutions	205
1963	Pharmaceutical Aspects of Drug Absorption	209
1964	Scientific Dosage Form Design	215
1965	Powder Technology of Solid Dosage Forms	227
1966	Pharmaceutical Coating	232
1967	Intermolecular Interactions of Solids in Pharmaceutical Solids	175
1968	Biophysical Basis for Dermatologic Formulation	182
1969	Pharmaceutical Parameters in Container Selection	162
1970	Complexation in Pharmaceutical Systems	124
1971	Drug Absorption Through the Gastrointestinal Barrier	172
1972	Improved Drug Activity Through Physicochemical Modification	142
1973	Recent Approaches to Drug Delivery Systems	151
1974	Parenteral Drug Delivery Systems	97
1975	Pharmaceutical Aspects of Solids	112
1976	Dosage Form Assessment: Physical and Biological Models	60
1977	Polymers	94
1978	Oral Administration of Drugs: Problems and Prospects	110
1979	Drug Metabolism; Implications in Product Development	78
1980	Drug Development in the 80's; Scale-up, Technology and Regulations	120
1981	Pharmaceutical Coating	125
1982	Solids Formulation: Precompressional Aspects	139
1983	Controlled and Targeted Drug Delivery Systems: Theory and Practice	138
1984	Design of Oral Dosage Forms Based on Physiological Considerations of the Gastrointestinal Tract	139
1985	The Use and Characterization of Polymers in Oral Dosage Forms	125
1986	Pharmaceutical Considerations in the Use of Peptides and Proteins	173
1987	Current Status and Future Directions of Transdermal Drug Delivery	150
1988	Design of Liquid Dosage Forms: Solutions and Dispersions	100
1989	Properties of Pharmaceutical Materials: Consequences for Processing and Performance of Solid Dosage Forms	100
1990	Challenges in the Development of Protein Drug Products	173
1991	Considerations in the Measurement and Control of Particles in Pharmaceuticals	145
1992	Pharmaceutical Excipients: Characterization, Functionality and Harmonization	162
1993	Development of Oral Dosage Forms for Poorly Bioavailable Drugs	148
1994	Stability, Instability and Product Quality: Mechanisms and Prediction	155
1995	Multi-Phase Systems for Oral and Parenteral Drug Delivery: Physical and Biopharmaceutical Aspects	100

Lemberger, and G. Zografi) have been elected president of the Academy of Pharmaceutical Sciences.

Four faculty members (G. Urdang, G. Sonnedecker, J. Parascandola, and J. Scarborough) and an adjunct faculty member (G. Higby), have served as the Director of the American Institute of the History of Pharmacy (AIHP), which was founded in Madison in 1941.

The Edward Kremers Professorship, a University of Wisconsin Chair, has been held by several faculty members in recognition of their distinguished service to the School and the field: Takeru Higuchi, 1964–66; Arthur H. Uhl, 1969–71; Louis W. Busse, 1977–78; David Perlman, 1979–80; Glenn Sonnedecker, 1981–86.

Charles J. Sih was named the first F. B. Power Professor of Pharmaceutical Chemistry in 1977; Daniel H. Rich became the WARF Ralph F. Hirschmann Professor in 1994; C. Richard Hutchinson was appointed Edward Leete Professor in 1995; and Robert W. Hammel became the William S. Apple Professor emeritus.

Named professorships and high-level administrative posts, by their nature, can recognize only the few. Many more members of the pharmacy faculty have earned awards and prizes in their field of expertise, when brought into comparison with their peers nationally, or internationally. As evidence in point, *Appendix 6* (p. 217) lists honors received during or following tenure at UW. The list admittedly is still incomplete—especially with regard to early faculty members—and it is somewhat selective (for example, election to fellowship in scholarly societies is not listed).[29] Although clinical faculty are not members of the graduate faculty, the research they conduct comes within the scope of this chapter and Appendix 6.

As another dimension that exemplifies faculty productivity and research interests, *Appendix 6.II* lists books written or edited and journals edited by faculty members, to the extent titles could be gathered for the present purpose.[30,31] Besides the activities and honors here put in the record, there were invited services by faculty members that imply recognition of research excellence: the refereeing of manuscripts and research proposals, the reviewing of books, the consulting services to governmental agencies and the pharmaceutical industry.

Nature and Impact of the Research. As the results of research reveal new areas for investigation and as they suggest new questions to investigators, the types and emphasis of the research work in an institution change. The research carried out in the School of Pharmacy during the past century has

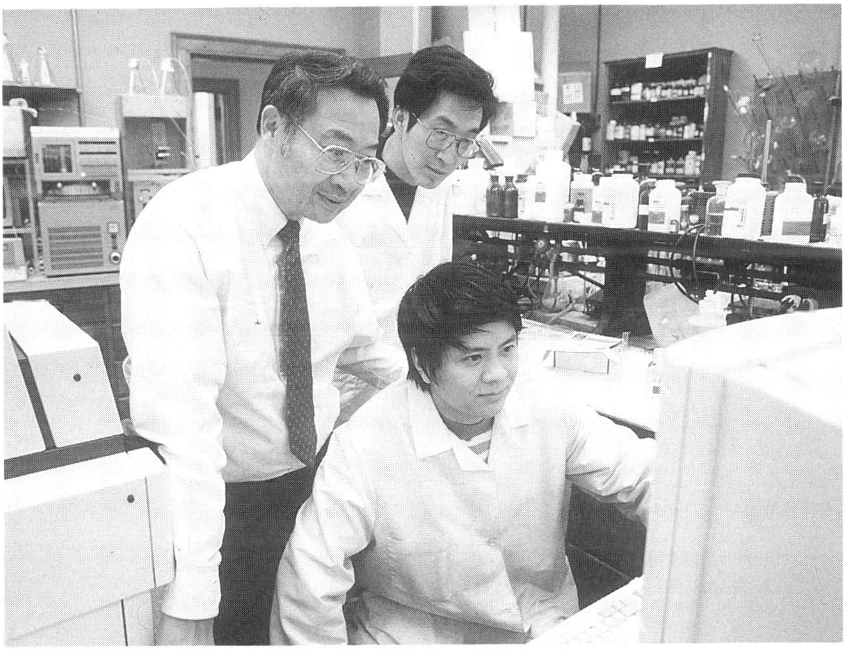

Pharmaceutical biochemistry became increasingly significant in the School during the 1960s, after Charles J. Sih (above left) joined the pharmacy faculty.

reflected such shifts. In many instances the faculty have initiated changes in direction that were later followed by workers elsewhere. An excellent example of such leadership is the development of "physical pharmacy," which is the physico-chemical study of pharmaceutical systems.

As an approach to investigating chemical and pharmaceutical problems the use of physical-chemical methods was not new, but their applications to pharmaceutical preparations had seldom been carried out systematically or with the aid of contemporaneous understanding of physical-chemical principles and methods of attack. For example, it had long been common practice to study the effect of temperature on the stability of pharmaceutical preparations, but in such studies other important variables (such as pH) were not controlled or measured, so that the experimental results were applicable merely to the particular instance, with no general inferences being possible. Physical pharmacy therefore constituted a new research point of view in pharmacy, and this approach, which was largely developed at Wisconsin in the 1950s, had a profound influence on the later views of how pharmaceutical systems should be studied and on the kinds of information that are needed.

Instead of presenting a decade-by-decade description of the research enterprise at the School of Pharmacy, the nature of the work is portrayed here by brief characterization of the faculty members' research contributions as revealed by their publications.[32] Those faculty are included who published sufficiently to have had a significant effect on the kinds of work being done at the School within the present scope, 1883 to 1983, leaving out of account recent work in progress. For each researcher, the dates of membership on the School faculty are given in parentheses.

Albrecht, Ralph M. (1979–85). Macrophage and platelet structure and function, using cell biology and microscopy techniques.

Amidon, Gordon L. (1971–82). His early work was on theoretical calculations of intermolecular forces in molecular complexes, enzyme-substrate complexes, and drug-receptor interactions. A later series dealt with solubilities of nonelectrolytes in polar solvents. His latest work at Wisconsin was on pro-drugs designed to make use of endogenous enzymes to achieve selective drug delivery. He left Wisconsin to join INTERx division of Merck Sharp & Dohme, and then became a faculty member at the University of Michigan.

Arndt, Jack R. (1961–77). Continuing education for pharmacists; program evaluation. He left Wisconsin for the University of Arizona.

Bardell, Eunice Bonow (1952–72). Pharmaceutical history, especially of Wisconsin.

Bass, Paul (1970–). Gastrointestinal pharmacology, including the mechanism of action of laxatives, gastric emptying times, GI transit times, and quantitative evaluation of GI contractile activity.

Blockstein, William L. (1964–91). Continuing education for pharmacists and other health professionals; health planning and pharmaceutical education; evaluation of continuing education programs.

Buckner, Carl K. (1970–87). Adrenergic pharmacology, including measurement of dissociation constants of ß-adrenergic receptor agonist interactions. Immunopharmacology, histamine release, and mediators of immediate hypersensitivity reactions. He left Wisconsin for industry, and in 1995 he joined the staff of the American Council on Pharmaceutical Education.

Busse, Louis W. (1940–78). In the 1950s he published in several areas of physical pharmacy. Particularly notable was a series of papers on the physics of tablet compression. Other papers described protective ointment bases, the spray-drying of drugs, and the heat sterilization of thermally labile pharmaceuticals. He was active in developing the extension services in pharmacy, and was in large part responsible for initiating the Land O' Lakes Conferences. In his position as Associate Dean he was able to stimulate research by supporting the appointment of able faculty and by attracting graduate students to the program.

Cannon, Joseph G. (1956–62). Synthesis of biologically active molecules, especially alkynes. He left Wisconsin to join the University of Iowa.

Carstensen, Jens T. (1968–95). Physical chemistry of dosage form design, production, and testing, the emphasis being on solid state dosage forms. Application of statistics to pharmaceutical problems (such as shelf-life estimates and powder blending); dissolution kinetics theory and technology; sedimentation kinetics of floculated suspensions; milling, mixing, and flow of granulations; and solid state decomposition of drugs and dosage forms constitute some of his research contributions.

Connors, Kenneth A. (1962–97). Organic analytical reactions, their catalysis, mechanisms, and applications; also kinetic methods for the analysis of mixtures; and the chemistry of molecular complexes, including cyclodextrin complexes.

Dickson, W. Michael (1974–80). Allocation of pharmacist's time and labor in community pharmacies.

Durant, Winston J. (1960–71). Hospital medication distribution systems and unit dose packaging. He left Wisconsin to join Becton Dickinson Co.

Ellison, Robert A. (1969–75). Organic synthesis, for example via 1,3-dithianes and alkyllithium reagents. Later work with chemistry of T–2 toxin.

Ericksen, Stuart P. (1960–65). Found methanol in human breath. Formulated theory of drug release from sustained action dosage forms. Also collaborated (with T. Higuchi) on tablet compression and (with S. M. Kupchan) on intramolecular catalysis of ester solvolysis. Left Wisconsin to join Allergan Pharmaceuticals.

Foye, William O. (1949–55). A synthetic medicinal chemist. Prepared derivatives and analogs of amino aldehydes, aminosalicylic acids, triazines, metal complexes of alloxan and functionalized aromatics.

Finger, Kenneth F. (1962–68). Studied effects of agonists on free fatty acid release. He was the first pharmacologist to join the faculty; he left Wisconsin to become Dean at the University of Florida.

Hammel, Robert W. (1958–90). His work dealt mainly with the economics of pharmacy practice, including prescription pricing, patterns of prescribing, pharmacy economic growth, and salaries. Other areas of interest were the attitudes of pharmacists and physicians toward the drug industry, unions, and associations; and legal aspects of pharmacy.

Hart, Phillip A. (1964–95). Primarily known for the application of nuclear magnetic resonance to the study of nucleoside and nucleotide conformation in solution by means of the nuclear Overhauser effect; he also used optical rotatory dispersion and circular dichroism measurements.

Higuchi, Takeru (1947–67). Trained as a physical chemist, he is widely regarded as "the father of physical pharmacy." This listing of areas in which he published while at Wisconsin is not exhaustive: physics of tablet compression; kinetics of drug decomposition (including chloramphenicol, procaine, epinephrine, thiamine, niacinamide, vitamin A, ascorbic acid); molecular complexes (a series describing hundreds of stability constant determinations); theory of drug release from heterogeneous matrices; nonaqueous acid-base chemistry; spectrophotometric titrations; ion-pair extraction equilibria; formation of amides in aqueous solution; solvate formation and dissolution rates; chlorination of amines;

thermodynamics of phase transitions; applications of chromatography. He directed the research of about 75 Ph.D. students at Wisconsin, and through collaboration with other faculty had an influence on the research of other groups. He played a part in establishing the Land O' Lakes Conferences, and served as first president of the Academy of Pharmaceutical Sciences. He had a strong influence on the conduct of pharmaceutical research and development in the drug industry. He left Wisconsin to join the faculty at the University of Kansas.

Higuchi, William I. (1959–62). Theoretical physical chemistry: drug release from ointments; kinetics of suspension aggregation; emulsion particle size changes; polymorphism and solubility. He left Wisconsin for the College of Pharmacy, University of Michigan; later he moved to the University of Utah.

Hutchinson, C. Richard (1975–). Biosynthesis of macrolide antibiotics, camptothecin, iridoids, and indole alkaloids.

Kirk, Kenneth W. (1972–75). Adult education theory applied to pharmacy continuing education; women pharmacy practitioners. He left Wisconsin for Purdue University.

Kremers, Edward (1891–1935). Primarily a plant chemist with special interests in volatile oils and the terpenes. He also published on topics in pharmaceutics, such as a systematization of types of dosage forms; and on pharmaceutical education. Perhaps his most influential work, however, was in the history of pharmacy, and his book on this subject in collaboration with G. Urdang (later editions revised by G. Sonnedecker) remains the standard text.

Kupchan, S. Morris (1957–69). A prolific investigator of biologically active products from plants. His work was systematic and thorough. Although not limited to these subjects, his published work included extensive studies of veratrum and buxus alkaloids, and a series reaching seventy papers (based on work while he was at Wisconsin) on tumor inhibitors from plants. A distinguishing feature of this series is that the fractionation and isolation of the constituents were guided at each stage by biological assays, resulting in the occasional isolation of important minor constituents that might have otherwise been overlooked. He left Wisconsin for the Department of Chemistry, University of Virginia.[33]

Lage, Gary C. (1973–79). Metabolism of digitalis compounds. He left Wisconsin to establish the toxicology program at the Philadelphia College of Pharmacy and Science.

Langenhan, Henry A. (1913–23). Properties and preparation of pharmaceuticals.

Lemberger, August P. (1953–69; 1980–91). Numerous subjects in physical pharmacy, such as kinetics of tropine ester hydrolyses, suspension viscosity, aggregation in emulsions and suspensions, and soybean lecithin films. In the 1960s he participated in the development of pharmacy extension services and in continuing education programs. He became Dean of the College of Pharmacy, University of Illinois, then returned to Wisconsin as Dean in 1980.

Mellon, William S. (1979–). Nature and cellular location of the biological receptor for 1,25-dihydroxyvitamin D3 and the disposition of the drug-receptor complex.

Morin, Robert (1971–73). Synthetic medicinal chemistry, especially of ß-lactam antibiotics. His research included prostaglandin and penicillin biosynthetic studies.

Mukerjee, Pasupati (1967–94). Association of molecules in solution, especially formation of micelles and their properties. His work combined theory and experiment with the aims of determining micellar structure and size distribution, establishing the polarity of micelle microenvironments (by means of spectroscopic probes), and measuring the distribution of solubilized species in the micelle core and mantle.

Nelson, Eino (1954–55). Physics of tablet compression; he took part (with L. W. Busse) in the construction of the first instrumented tablet machine.

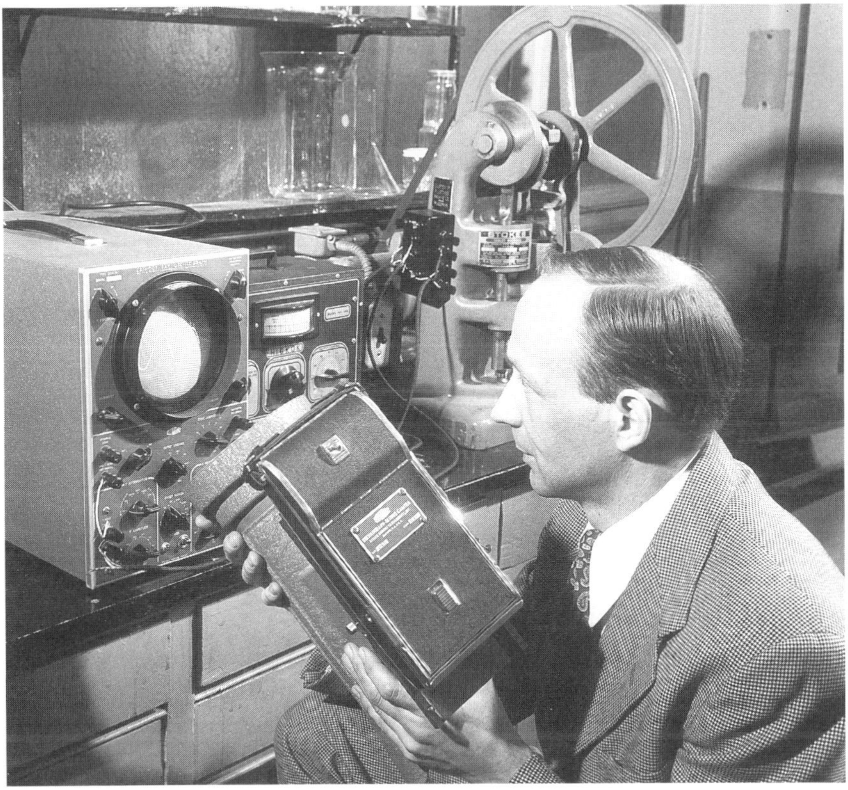

An instrumented tabletting machine to study the physics of compression (c. 1954) was an early expression of "physical pharmacy," a field pioneered by the School. An early doctoral candidate in the field, Eino Nelson (shown above), became a nationally prominent pharmacokineticist.

Northrop, Dexter B. (1971–). Enzyme kinetics with contributions in two areas: isolation, properties, and analytical uses of antibiotic transferases; and the interpretation of kinetic isotope effects in enzyme-catalyzed reactions.

Ohvall, Richard A. (1964–71). Vocational planning of pharmacy students; women pharmacists' practice patterns. He left Wisconsin to become Dean at Ferris State College, then Dean at the University of Oregon.

Parascandola, John L. (1969–83). History of drug use, and history of pharmacology; of particular interest are studies on the biochemist L. J. Henderson, early structure-activity relationships, and receptor theory of drug action. He left Wisconsin to to become Chief of the History of Medicine Division, National Library of Medicine.

Parks, Lloyd M. (1937–56). Plant chemistry, especially of sabadilla alkaloids. He left Wisconsin to become the Dean at Ohio State University.

Perlman, David (1967–80). Fermentation processes, with extensive contributions on microbial transformations, peptide antibiotics, antibiotics as enzyme substrates, tissue culture as an experimental tool, microbial production of vitamin B12 antimetabolites, L-sorbose bioconversion. His review articles on these topics and on the fermentation industries were valuable. During his seven-year period of service as Dean of the School he pursued his active research program, and his research productivity continued even during his long terminal illness.

Perrin, John H. (1962–73). Study of drug aggregation and protein binding by circular dichroism-optical rotatory dispersion; absorption of amine salts in the stomach; enhancement of drug absorption by competitive protein binding.

Peterson, Richard E. (1975–). Toxicology, particularly the distribution, metabolism, and elimination of chlorinated hydrocarbons in mammals and fish.

Porter, William R. (1978–85). Stability of solution dosage forms; chemistry and metabolism of anticoagulant drugs; metabolism and pharmacokinetics of sulfur-containing drugs and toxicants. He left to join Abbott Laboratories.

Power, Frederick B. (1883–92). Plant chemistry, with most of his work being accomplished after he left Wisconsin. He carried out phytochemical studies of many common fruits, berries, and seeds, including grape, apple, peach, pumpkin, watermelon, and wheat; and studied the constituents of nutmeg, cotton, jalap, ipomea, taraxacum, clover, sarsaparilla, hops, and eriodictyon.

Rich, Daniel H. (1970–). Peptide synthesis and mechanism of action, especially cyclic peptides and protease inhibitors. His work includes synthetic methods, synthesis and conformational studies of tentoxin and chlamydocin, pepstatin inhibition of carboxyl proteases, bestatin inhibition of amino peptidases and synthesis of substrates and inhibitors for vitamin K-dependent carboxylase.

Richtmann, William O. (1898–1902; 1919–47). Pharmaceutical preparations; American species of verbena.

Robinson, Joseph R. (1966–). His early work was on physical organic chemical investigations of ester solvolyses and empirical models for linear free energy relationships; he also contributed (in part with S. P. Eriksen) to the theory of sustained release dosage forms. In the 1970s he initiated studies on drug absorption, distribution, and elimination in the eye, with experimental evaluation of the effects of tear turnover, protein binding, transcorneal permeation mechanisms, and vehicle effects.

Rudy, Thomas A. (1971–). Two areas have been investigated: the sites of action of the antinociceptive effect of morphine and other narcotics; and central nervous system mechanisms of temperature regulation and fever.

Sih, Charles J. (1960–). His research has made extensive use of microbial transformations of organic compounds. In the 1960s he developed methods for microbial conversions of steroids, and studied the mechanism of steroid hydroxylation. In the 1970s biosynthetic routes to the prostaglandins were described. He has published synthetic or biosynthetic methods for many other compounds, including L-dopa, leukotriene A, adriamycinone, arachidonic acid, and strigol.

Smissman, Edward E. (1955–60). Organic synthesis and reaction mechanisms, for example the quasi-Favorskii rearrangement, the Prins reaction, and the acid-catalyzed rearrangement of phenylethynylcarbinols. He left Wisconsin to join the University of Kansas.

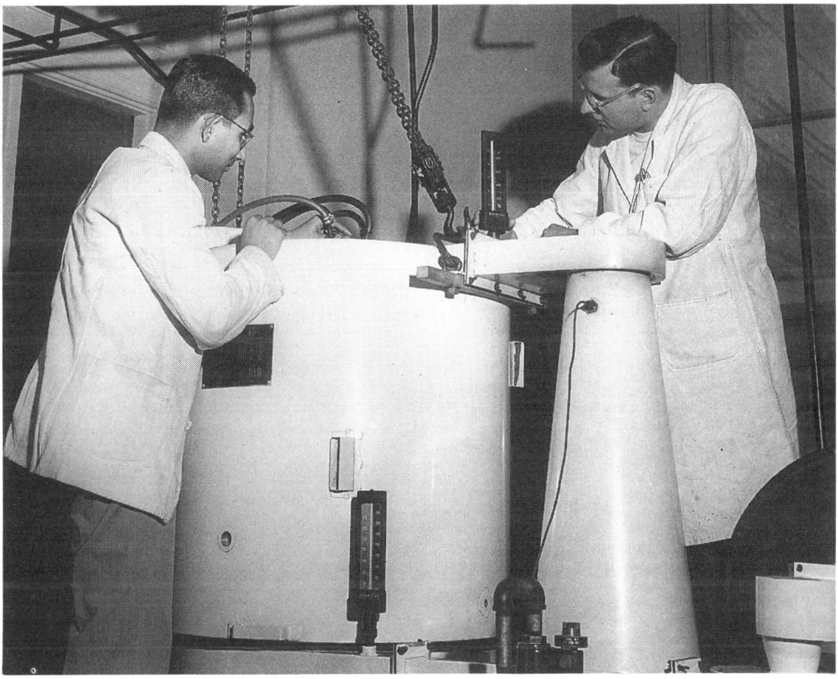

Spray-drying techniques in the manufacture of pharmaceuticals became a fruitful line of research at the School. Two graduate students, Mohit C. Gupta and Robert Schleif, are shown preparing an experiment, about 1952.

Sonnedecker, Glenn A. (1952–86). History of pharmacy, with special attention to American pharmacy: including articles on USP and NF history, nineteenth-century pharmaceutical education, the rise of drug manufacturers in America, legalization of drug standards, and more general topics, such as the evolution of the concept of opiate addiction. He also helped initiate graduate study of the social aspects of the profession.

Stieb, Ernst W. (1958–67). American pharmacy's history and, especially, the history of drug quality standards and drug adulteration in Britain and Canada. He left Wisconsin for the University of Toronto.

Svarstad, Bonnie L. (1975–). Social issues in pharmacy and drug use, including physician-pharmacist-patient communication, and patient non-compliance with drug regimens.

Swintosky, Joseph V. (1948–53). Solids and solid dosage forms. He played a seminal role by introducing T. Higuchi to A. H. Uhl. After leaving Wisconsin he led a dosage form research group at Smith Kline and French Laboratories, and later became Dean of the University of Kentucky College of Pharmacy.

Thielke, Thomas S. (1970–). Hospital pharmacy administration: computerization, productivity measurements, drug education.

Uhl, Arthur H. (1930–31; 1935–71). His research was in plant chemistry, often in collaboration with L. M. Parks. However, his influence on pharmaceutical research came through his role as Dean of the School; in this role he built a strong research faculty and helped them develop financial support for research.

Urdang, George (1947–52). He collaborated with E. Kremers on the book *A History of Pharmacy* (1940) and served as the founding Director of the American Institute of the History of Pharmacy even before he was made a member of the faculty. His contributions treated many aspects of pharmaceutical history, such as the development of the pharmaceutical literature, retail pharmacy as the origin of the pharmaceutical industry, biographical essays (e.g., on Martin Klaproth, Edward Kremers, Carl Scheele, Edward Parrish), pharmacopeias as witnesses of world history, the entry of chemical entities into pharmacopeias, reflections of pharmacy in creative literature, the history of pharmacy in Germany and in the United States.

Wakeman, Nellie A. (1913–46). Pigments of flowering plants; chemistry of thymoquinone.

Weinswig, Melvin H. (1969–). Drug abuse education and prevention; continuing education for pharmacy practitioners, detailmen, and non-practicing pharmacists; evaluation of telelecture and audiocassette continuing education courses.

Welling, Peter G. (1972–84). A very prolific publisher of bioavailability and pharmacokinetic studies, often in collaboration with medical practitioners. Many papers dealt with drug absorption and elimination kinetics in patients with impaired renal function. Another series explored the effects of food and fluid uptake on gastrointestinal drug absorption.

Windheuser, John J. (1963–72). Drug analysis.

19. These counts are based on graduates' names, and therefore may not be accurate. Surely the most interesting name among all graduates is Nevada Marie Hanson Huntington Windemuth (Mrs. Higgins), M.S. (1934), Ph.D. (1938).
20. Figure 5.3 was constructed from the data on School of Pharmacy faculty members (Appendix 2).
21. This brief sketch of some of the notable contributions to the development of the graduate and research programs of the School is obviously very selective and is meant to identify those figures who played significant seminal roles. Important research contributions have been made by many other members of the faculty during the more mature stages of development of each curricular area, as described on p. 155.
22. This account is based largely upon an unpublished paper, "The Pharmaceutical Experiment Station in Madison, Wisconsin, 1913–1933," by Sami K. Hamarneh (undated, but about 1957), KRF.
23. The Pure Food and Drug Act had been passed in 1906 partly in response to this situation. See, e.g., *The Early Years of Federal Food and Drug Control* (Madison, 1982), 60 pp.
24. Even into the 1980s, former students of Prof. Kremers recalled their experiences in this setting. Paul J. Jannke (Ph.D., 1938), Professor-Emeritus, University of Connecticut, described the harvest, transportation, and distillation of plant drugs, a large still being installed in the space between Sterling Hall and the Chemistry Building. (Personal communication with K. A. Connors, February 1981.)
25. KRF, C31(a)I, University of Wisconsin, 1883–1933. In the actual budget for this year, Kremers is allotted $500 as Director of the Experiment Station; and he received a salary of $3000 as Director of the Department. In 1917 the legislature increased the annual appropriation to $5,000, at least in part as a war measure.
26. Clarence Sondern (Ph.D., 1933) recalled working in the garden, which was near Picnic Point west of University Bay Drive. (Personal communication with Glenn Sonnedecker, December 29, 1981.)
27. Researchers in the School of Pharmacy have been greatly benefitted by the support of numerous staff members whose commitment to the School constitutes a valuable research facility. For example, graduate alumni of the 1950–80 period were often indebted to support personnel whose periods of service in the School have been extensive: secretaries Lois Lane, Billie Hubacher, and Linda Frei; and personnel responsible for supplies, purchasing, and facilities: Mern Kier, Harry Alexander, Norm Gjerde, Ken Berg, Bob Aylesworth, and Jerry Kozel.
28. During the same week of June 14–19, 1981, the School of Pharmacy was the host to the annual Pharmaceutics Graduate Student Research Meeting, with 140 persons from eleven schools of pharmacy; Ms. Sharon Laughlin of Wisconsin organized the symposium.
29. An exception should be made here to note that George Zografi was elected to membership in the prestigious Institute of Medicine of the National Academy of Sciences (1989). Although the present focus is on recognition for outstanding scholarly contributions, note also should be taken of service so exception-

al as educators that at least four of the pharmacy faculty received national or all-university honors: The AACP Distinguished Educator award has been conferred on George Zografi (1989) and on Kenneth A. Connors (1995); the UW Kiekhofer Memorial Teaching Award has been conferred on August P. Lemberger (1957) and the UW–Madison/Milwaukee Amoco Distinguished Teaching Award has been conferred on Joseph R. Robinson (1980).

30. There is some ambiguity in deciding what a book is for the purpose of this listing. For example, a part of a book is not a book, hence chapters, some of them quite long enough to be books, have not been listed. Also omitted are numerous lengthy papers published as monographs, but having the essential character of research articles.

31. Compiled from the University of Wisconsin–Madison Memorial Library Union Catalog and *Books in Print, 1980–1981*. Article reprints, loose-leaf texts, and taped lectures and notes are not included. Also omitted are chapters in books, separately printed research articles, and theses (see note 30).

32. And, it must be added, as interpreted by the author of this chapter, who is responsible for the evaluations of research significance and impact.

33. It is interesting that Professor Kupchan signed his papers "Department of Pharmaceutical Chemistry, University of Wisconsin" rather than "School of Pharmacy, University of Wisconsin".

Appendices

Appendix 1

Deans of the First Century (1883–1983)

Biographical essays by John Parascandola

DURING its first century the School had six chief administrators, called Chairman or Director until the title Dean was authorized in 1950 when the School became independent of the College of Letters and Science. All but one were graduates in pharmacy. All held a Ph.D. in some branch of pharmaceutical science, two from German universities and three of the other four from the University of Wisconsin. All were born and reared east of the Mississippi. Portraits that illustrate the following essays were photographed during their tenure as deans.

Frederick Belding Power (1853–1927)

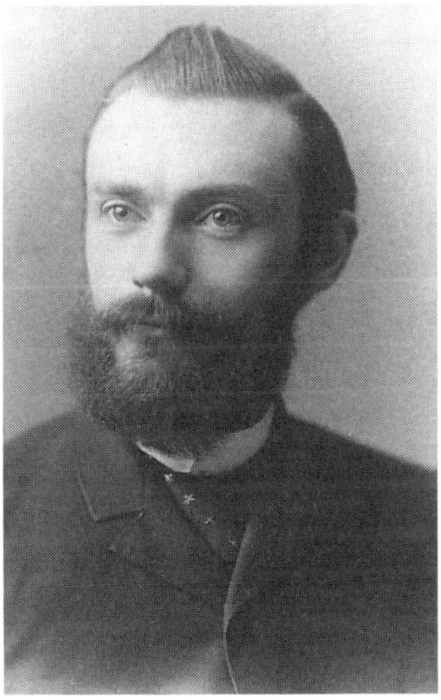
Frederick Belding Power, 1883–1892

Frederick B. Power was born in Hudson, New York on March 4, 1853, the son of Thomas and Caroline (Belding) Power. He obtained his early education at a private school and at the Hudson Academy. Power worked for several years in a local pharmacy and briefly in a Chicago pharmacy before accepting a position in the establishment of a notably prominent pharmacist in Philadelphia, Edward Parrish. Although his employer died shortly thereafter, Power continued to work for the Parrish firm and also attended the Philadelphia College of Pharmacy, from which he graduated in 1874. After two more years with the Parrish firm, Power decided to undertake graduate study in chemistry and the pharmaceutical sciences in Germany. He received his Ph.D. in 1880 from the University of Strassburg, where he served as assistant to the noted pharmacognosist Friedrich Flückiger.

Upon returning to the United States, Power taught analytical chemistry at his alma mater, the Philadelphia College of Pharmacy, until 1883, when he received the call to the University of Wisconsin to serve as the first director of its newly created Department of Pharmacy. A gentle, kindly man and an untiring worker devoted to research and scholarship, Power guided the Wisconsin pharmacy program through its infant years and placed it on a sound scientific footing.

In 1892, he resigned his position at Wisconsin to become scientific director of the chemical laboratories of Fritzsche Brothers in Passaic, New Jersey. Tragedy struck the following year when his wife, the former Mary Von Loan Meigs, died two weeks after giving birth to their third child.

Power moved to London in 1896 when his lifelong friend and fellow classmate at the Philadelphia College of Pharmacy, Henry Wellcome, established the Wellcome Chemical Research Laboratories there and appointed Power as director. He returned to the United States in 1914, and two years later became head of the Phytochemistry Laboratory of the United States Department of Agriculture in Washington, D.C., a position he held until his death on March 26, 1927.

Power's research interests were centered in the field of phytochemistry. He added significantly to our knowledge of plant chemistry by isolating and purifying numerous constituents from a host of different plant substances (e.g., nutmeg, cotton, fruits), and by determining the chemical structures of many of these constituents. Probably his best known work was his research on chaulmoogra oil, a traditional remedy for leprosy in the Orient which entered Western medicine in the nineteenth century. Power and his coworkers at the Wellcome Laboratories isolated two new fatty acids, chaulmoogric and hydnocarpic acids, from the oil. They also determined the structures of these compounds, although the formulas assigned have since been modified. Sulfones have since replaced chaulmoogra oil in the treatment of leprosy.

Among the honors awarded to Power during his lifetime were the Hanbury Gold Medal (1913), the Flückiger Gold Medal (1922), the Ebert Prize (three times) and election to the National Academy of Sciences (1924).

• • •

For further information, see John Parascandola, "Frederick Belding Power," *Dictionary of Scientific Biography*, vol. 11, pp. 120–121; Max Phillips, "Frederick Belding Power, Most Distinguished American Phytochemist," *Journal of Chemical Education*, 31(1954):258–261; and Ivor Griffith, "A Half Century of Research in Plant Chemistry: A Chronological Record of the Scientific Contributions of Frederick Belding Power," *American Journal of Pharmacy*, 96(1924):605–613. The Kremers Reference Files of the F. B. Power Pharmaceutical Library, University of Wisconsin, Madison, contain a significant amount of Power manuscript materials, including correspondence of Power and an unpublished biographical memoir by his daughter.

Edward Kremers (1865–1941)

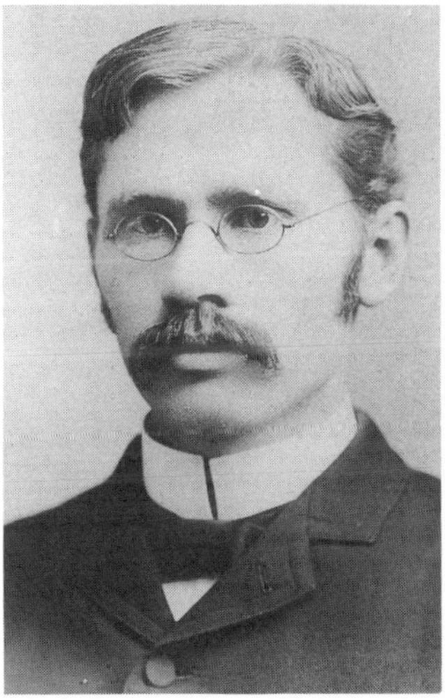

Edward Kremers, 1892–1935

Edward Kremers was born in Milwaukee, Wisconsin on February 23, 1865, the son of German immigrants Gerhard and Elise (Kamper) Kremers. His upbringing was steeped in Germanic tradition, as he attended schools oriented toward German culture and apprenticed in the Milwaukee "Apotheke" of German-born Louis Lotz. After spending the 1884–85 academic year at the Philadelphia College of Pharmacy, Kremers returned to his native state to complete his Ph.G. degree in 1886 in the recently established pharmacy program at the University of Wisconsin. A desire for further education led him to take the B.Sc. degree in General Science at Wisconsin in 1888 and then on to advanced studies in Germany, earning a Ph.D. from the University of Goettingen in 1890 for research on terpenes under Otto Wallach.

Kremers had become well acquainted with Frederick B. Power as a student at Wisconsin and as his assistant for the 1886–87 academic year. Upon the completion of his studies in Germany, Kremers accepted an invitation from Power to become an instructor in pharmacy at the University of Wisconsin in the fall of 1890. When Power left Wisconsin in 1892, Kremers succeeded his mentor as director of the pharmacy program.

Edward Kremers was a dedicated reformer committed to improving the status of the profession of pharmacy. At Wisconsin he introduced a number of innovative programs that had an impact on the national scene, most notably the first B.Sc. in pharmacy and the first Ph.D. in pharmaceutical specialties to be offered in this country. More than 50 Ph.D. students received their training under Kremers, and many went on to positions of leadership in American pharmacy. He was also responsible for the creation of the Pharmaceutical Experiment Station in Madison.

Kremers' humanistic interests found their major outlet in his historical work. He was responsible for introducing instruction in history of pharmacy and history of chemistry at Wisconsin in the early years of this century, was a co-founder of the American Pharmaceutical Association's Section on Historical Pharmacy (1904) and later the American Institute of the History of Pharmacy (1941), and was instrumental in bringing George

Urdang to Madison in 1939. Urdang drew upon the vast historical collections of Kremers in serving as the principal author of the Kremers-Urdang *History of Pharmacy* (1940).

Kremers' research interests, and those of his students, centered largely around phytochemistry. On two occasions (1897, 1900) he received the Ebert Prize of the American Pharmaceutical Association for his research. Volatile oils was a field of special emphasis for Kremers, and in 1900 the first edition of his English translation of Gildemeister and Hoffmann's classic book, *The Volatile Oils*, appeared.

An active participant in several professional societies, Kremers served as president of the American Conference of Pharmaceutical Faculties and of the Wisconsin Pharmaceutical Association, and as honorary president of the American Pharmaceutical Association, the National Association of Boards of Pharmacy and the American Institute of the History of Pharmacy. He also served on the Wisconsin State Board of Pharmacy and the United States Pharmacopeia Revision Committee, and as Chairman of the Scientific Section of the American Pharmaceutical Association. In addition, he served for a number of years as editor of *The Pharmaceutical Review* and *Pharmaceutical Archives*. Among the honors that he received during his lifetime, in addition to those already mentioned, were the Remington Honor Medal (1930) and an honorary Sc.D. degree from the University of Michigan (1913).

An outspoken, aggressive fighter who refused to compromise his ideals, Kremers naturally antagonized some of his colleagues at times. He also had many friends and admirers, but few could penetrate his austere dignity to know him intimately. A man of astonishing intellect and energy, with a broad range of interests, Kremers left an indelible mark on the Wisconsin School of Pharmacy, which he headed for 43 years until his retirement in 1935. He died in Madison on July 9, 1941, at the age of 76.

• • •

For further information, see George Urdang, "Edward Kremers (1965–1941): Reformer of American Pharmaceutical Education," *American Journal of Pharmaceutical Education*, 11(1947):631–658; George Urdang, "Obituary: Dr. Edward Kremers," *Science*, 94(1941):293–294; and Glenn Sonnedecker, "Pharmacy Educators of the Past: Edward Kremers," *AACP News*, vol. 4., no. 8, August 1976, p. 126. The Edward Kremers Papers, consisting of 21 boxes of correspondence, notes, memorabilia, etc., are housed in the Archives Division of the State Historical Society of Wisconsin in Madison. The Kremers Reference Files of the F. B. Power Pharmaceutical Library, University of Wisconsin–Madison, also contain a voluminous amount of correspondence and other materials by and/or related to Kremers.

Arthur Hoyt Uhl (1900–1979)

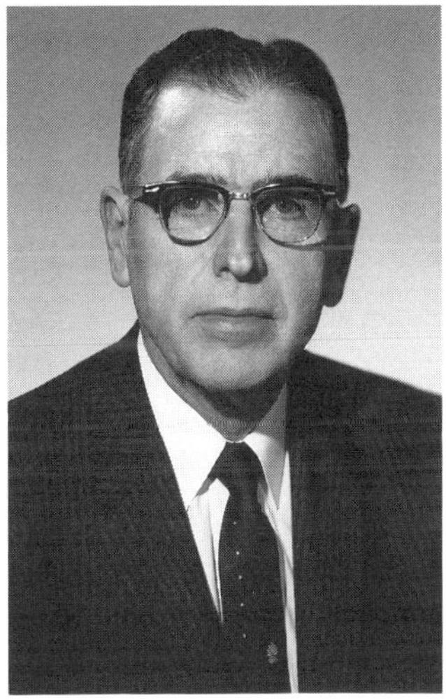

Arthur Hoyt Uhl, 1935–1968

Arthur H. Uhl was born in Galesville, Wisconsin, on July 31, 1900, the son of Philip and Sarah Susan (Hoyt) Uhl. After spending his youth on his parents' farm and in the Galesville school system, he entered the University of Wisconsin in 1919. Uhl received the Ph.G. diploma in 1921, and after two years of practical drugstore experience became registered in 1923. He returned to the University for further education, receiving B.Sc. (1926) and M.S. (1927) degrees in pharmacy.

After teaching pharmacy at Valparaiso University from 1927 to 1929, Uhl returned to Wisconsin again to continue his graduate studies, obtaining his Ph.D. degree in pharmacy under Edward Kremers in 1930. He remained on the Wisconsin faculty with the title of research associate until Kremers retired in 1935, whereupon Uhl became assistant professor of pharmacy and Kremers' successor as director of the pharmacy program. Uhl rose through the ranks to become associate professor in 1937 and professor in 1939. When the School of Pharmacy became an autonomous administrative unit in 1950, he was appointed its first dean, a position he resigned in 1968. He continued on the faculty until his retirement in 1970.

Uhl presided over a period of tremendous expansion in the history of the School of Pharmacy. The faculty grew from three in 1935 to a professional group of about 24 in 1968. The physical facilities of the School were significantly expanded during his deanship, especially through the completion in 1955 of a four-story pharmacy addition to the Chemistry Building. Student enrollment also increased several-fold during the Uhl years.

Possessing a remarkable ability to recognize and nurture talent, Uhl built a strong faculty which assured a continued leadership role for Wisconsin in American pharmaceutical education. He promoted the development of new fields, such as physical pharmacy and historical and social studies of pharmacy, making the School a pioneer in these areas. His capacity for leadership was recognized by the American Pharmaceutical Association in 1965 when it awarded him the Research Achievement Award for stimulation of research.

Although active at the national level, for example as President of the American Association of Colleges of Pharmacy and as Honorary President of the American Pharmaceutical Association, Uhl's primary commitment was to Wisconsin pharmacy. He served as President and Chairman of the Board of the Wisconsin Pharmaceutical Association, and was named Wisconsin Pharmacist of the Year in 1960.

Uhl shared Kremers' interest in the history of pharmacy, although, unlike his mentor, he did not directly contribute to historical research and writing. He was one of the founders of the American Institute of the History of Pharmacy and served as President (1941–55) and as Chairman of the Council (1955–71). Uhl was also instrumental in creating the first American chair in the history of pharmacy at the Wisconsin in 1947.

A friendly, compassionate man, Uhl had great rapport with his students, and was extremely popular among the pharmacists of the state. He died December 29, 1979, in Tucson, Arizona, and was returned to his beloved hometown of Galesville for burial.

• • •

For further information, see Louis Busse, Kenneth Connors, Robert Hammel, and Glenn Sonnedecker, "Arthur Hoyt Uhl," *American Journal of Pharmaceutical Education*, 44(1980):209; [Ernst Stieb], "A Quarter Century of Leadership, 1935–1960: Arthur H. Uhl, Twenty-five Eventful Years," *School of Pharmacy Bulletin*, University of Wisconsin Extension Division, May 1960, pp. 10–12; [Glenn Sonnedecker], "An AIHP Founder: A. H. Uhl (1900–1979)," *Pharmacy in History*, 22(1980):47–48. The Kremers Reference Files of the F. B. Power Pharmaceutical Library, University of Wisconsin, Madison contains a significant amount of manuscript materials (letters, lecture notes, etc.) related to Uhl. The transcript of a tape-recorded interview with Uhl concerning his career at Wisconsin is on deposit in the University of Wisconsin Archives in Madison.

David S. Perlman (1920–1980)

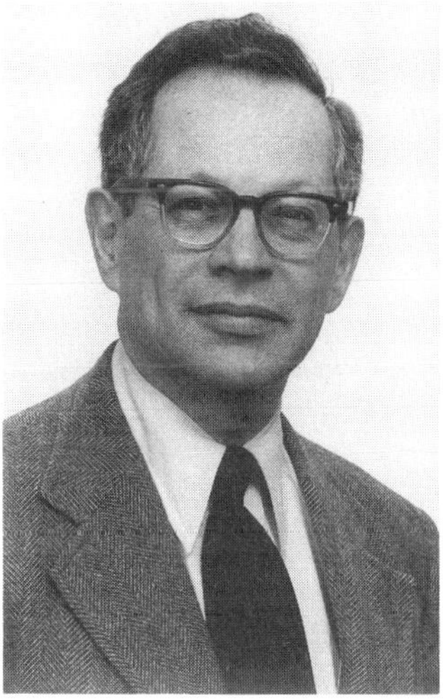

David Perlman, 1968–1975

David Perlman was born in Madison, Wisconsin, on February 6, 1920, the son of Selig and Eva (Shaber) Perlman. His father was a distinguished professor of economics at the University of Wisconsin. After receiving his primary and secondary education in the Madison schools, Perlman entered the University of Wisconsin, where he earned three degrees, B.A. (1941), M.S. (1943) and Ph.D. (1945). His doctoral dissertation in biochemistry involved fermentation studies under the guidance of Professor Marvin Johnson.

After receiving his doctorate, Perlman spent the next two decades as a research scientist in the pharmaceutical industry. After brief stints at Hoffman-LaRoche and Merck, he joined the staff of the Squibb Institute for Medical Research in 1947, and remained there until he accepted the position of professor of pharmaceutical biochemistry at the University of Wisconsin School of Pharmacy in 1967. A year later, upon the retirement of Arthur Uhl, Perlman became dean of the School. In 1975, he gave up the deanship to return to full-time teaching and research, remaining on the Wisconsin faculty until his death on January 29, 1980.

Perlman was a productive scientist who managed to keep a very active research program going even throughout the years of his deanship. His research interests centered around the fermentation biochemistry of antibiotics, steroids and vitamins. He was the author of nearly 300 scientific papers, about 75 professional papers, the editor of 27 books and the holder of 28 U.S. patents.

An active participant in professional organizations, Perlman held many society posts during his career, including serving as Chairman of the Division of Microbial Chemistry and Technology of the American Chemical Society, as Chairman of the Fermentation Division of the American Society for Microbiology, and as President of the American Society for Microbiology Foundation. He also served on the editorial board of five journals.

During Perlman's tenure as dean, the School of Pharmacy continued to expand its student body, faculty and facilities. Perlman placed a strong emphasis on excellence in research. The early part of his administration was troubled by the controversy over his appointment (opposed by many pharmacists of the state because of his lack of a pharmacy background) and by the height of the Vietnam antiwar movement on campus, culminating in the bombing of the Army Mathematics Research Center (which caused extensive damage to the adjacent Pharmacy Building).

Perlman devoted himself with tremendous energy and intensity to his work, spending long hours at his desk and laboratory bench. Even his battle of two and one-half years with cancer did not diminish his enthusiasm and dedication, and he was still conducting classes until the month before his death. A man who seldom relaxed, Perlman approached his leisure interests with the same intensity that he gave to his professional work.

During his lifetime, he received numerous honors, including the Marvin Johnson Research Award (1977), the Fisher Scientific Award in Applied and Environmental Microbiology (1979), the Charles Thom Award for Research in Applied Microbiology (1979) and the Pasteur Award for Applied Microbiology (1979). He was also elected to the rank of Fellow in the New York Academy of Sciences, the American Academy of Microbiology, and the Academy of Pharmaceutical Sciences.

• • •

For further information, see "David Perlman, 1920–1980," in *Fermentation:Science and Technology with a Future* (*Biotechnology and Bioengineering*, vol. 22, suppl. 1), ed. by Allen Laskin, Michael Flickinger and Elmer Garden, Jr. (New York: John Wiley and Sons, 1980), pp. 1–3; Asger Langlykke, "Obituary: David Perlman," *ASM News*, 46(1980):215–216; and William Blockstein, "David Perlman," *American Journal of Pharmaceutical Education*, 44(1980):210. The Kremers References Files of the F. B. Power Pharmaceutical Library, University of Wisconsin–Madison, contain a small amount of manuscript material related to Perlman.

George Zografi (1936–)

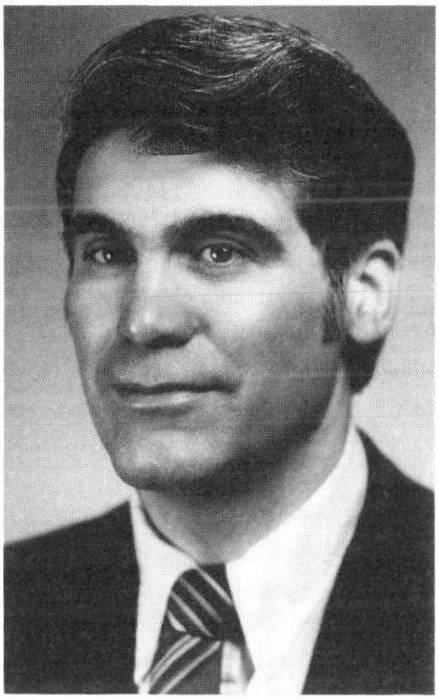

George Zografi, 1975–1980

George Zografi was born in New York City on March 13, 1936, the son of Elias and Parashgeva (Papasotir) Zografi. His father was a pharmacist, and Zografi decided to follow in his footsteps, earning his B.Sc. in pharmacy from his father's alma mater, the Columbia University College of Pharmacy, in 1956. He then embarked upon graduate studies, earning his M.S. in 1958 and his Ph.D. in 1960 from the University of Michigan College of Pharmacy for work in pharmaceutics.

From 1960 to 1964 he was assistant professor of pharmaceutics at Columbia, moving in the latter year to Michigan to fill the same post. Zografi was promoted to associate professor in 1967, and spent the 1970–71 year as Pfeiffer Memorial Fellow of the American Foundation for Pharmaceutical Education, conducting research at the University of Utrecht in the Netherlands. In 1972 he joined the faculty of the University of Wisconsin School of Pharmacy as professor of pharmaceutics. He succeeded David Perlman as Dean of the School in 1975 and served until 1980, when he elected to step down from the position to return to full-time teaching and research.

Zografi's research has focused on the design and evaluation of dosage forms, with an emphasis on the surface chemistry of pharmaceutical and biological systems. His scientific publications have dealt with such topics as lipid monomolecular films as models of biological membranes and the water vapor sorption and wettability of pharmaceutical solids.

Zografi has been an active participant in professional affairs. His contributions to professional organizations include service as president of the Academy of Pharmaceutical Sciences and of the American Association of Colleges of Pharmacy and as chairman of the Section of Teachers of Pharmacy of the American Association of Colleges of Pharmacy and of the Basic Pharmaceutics Section of the Academy of Pharmaceutical Sciences. His honors include an honorary Doctor of Science degree from the Columbia University College of Pharmaceutical Sciences (1976); the Volwiler Research Achievement Award (1996) and Distinguished Educator Award (1989)—the only person ever selected by the AACP to receive both; election to the Institute of Medicine of the National Academy of Sciences (1989); the Rho Chi Lecture Award (1997), a Distinguished Alumnus Award from the University of Michigan College of Pharmacy (1980), and a Fellowship in the Academy of Pharmaceutical Sciences.

A likable and easily approachable individual, Zografi's style of leadership involved keeping a relatively low profile as dean. Major accomplishments of his administration included a significant expansion of the clinical pharmacy program and the creation of the minority affairs program for the School.

• • •

For further information, see George Cocolas, "Meet the President," *Am. J. Pharm., Edu.* 47 (1983): 201–203, and "George Zografi Selected Dean of the University of Wisconsin School of Pharmacy," *Wisconsin Pharmacist*, 44 (1975):214.

August Paul Lemberger (1926–)

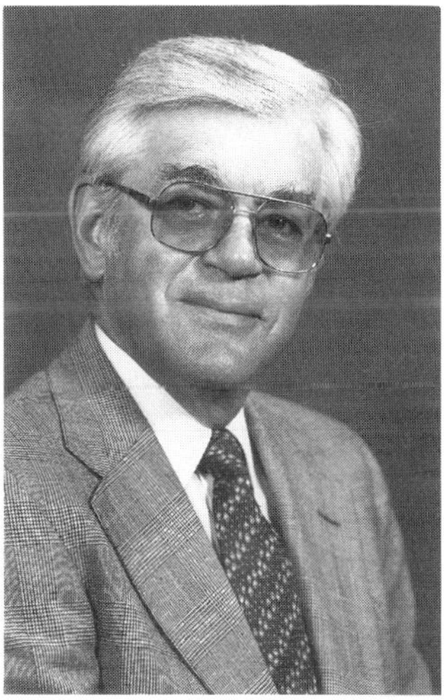

August Paul Lemberger, 1980–1991

August Lemberger was born in Milwaukee, Wisconsin, on January 25, 1926, the son of Max and Celia (Gehl) Lemberger. It was through the influence and encouragement of his father, a prominent Milwaukee pharmacist, that Lemberger decided to pursue a career in pharmacy. He entered the University of Wisconsin School of Pharmacy in 1943, but was called into military service the following year. He served in the United States Army from 1944 to 1946, when he was discharged with the rank of First Lieutenant. Returning to the University, he completed his B.Sc. degree in pharmacy in 1948, then continued on to receive his Ph.D. in 1952 for work in pharmaceutics.

Lemberger spent the next year as a senior chemist at Merck and Company, then returned to Wisconsin to join the faculty as instructor in pharmacy in 1953. He moved up through the ranks to assistant professor in 1955, associate professor in 1957, and professor in 1963. From 1965–69 he also served as coordinator of Extension Services in Pharmacy. Lemberger left Wisconsin in 1969 to become dean of the University of Illinois College of Pharmacy, but returned again to accept the deanship at the Wisconsin School of Pharmacy when George Zografi stepped down from the post in 1980.

Lemberger's effectiveness and popularity as a teacher earned him the Kiekhofer Teaching Award of the University of Wisconsin in 1957. His research has been in the area of physical pharmacy with special interest in polyphase systems and surface films.

His extensive professional service includes terms as president of the Academy of Pharmaceutical Sciences, vice president of the American Council on Pharmaceutical Education and of Rho Chi Society, and chairman of the Council of Deans and of the Teachers of Pharmacy Section of the American Association of Colleges of Pharmacy. His honors include the Kiekhofer Memorial Teaching Award from UW (1957), the Wisconsin Pharmaceutical Association Distinguished Service Award (1969), a University of Wisconsin Citation of Merit (1977), the Honorary Presidency of the American Pharmaceutical Association (1996–97); and a Fellowship in the Academy of Pharmaceutical Sciences and in the American Association for the Advancement of Science.

Lemberger brought a friendly, deliberate style to the deanship, a steadying influence during a period of ferment in professional programs of pharmaceutical education. In guiding the School to its first professional doctorate program (Pharm.D.), Lemberger made it a central principle to do so without compromising the School's traditional commitment to science and scholarship. He retired from the deanship and faculty in June 1991.

• • •

For further information, see "Pharmacy Professor Receives Kiekhofer Teaching Award," *Wisconsin Druggist*, 25 (5) (May 1957):8; "Dr. August P. Lemberger," *Drug Topics*, 104 (14) (July 18, 1960):32; and "Dr. Lemberger Named Dean," *Illinois Pharmacist*, 33 (3) (March 1969):125.

Part-time Administrators Appointed by the Deans

As the School grew and the University became more complex, selected faculty members were appointed by successive Deans to help administer the affairs of the School as a part-time, temporary assignment. The *Associate Deans* have been: Louis W. Busse (1950–68), Melvin Weinswig (1970–75), Kenneth A. Connors (1975–76), Bonnie L. Svarstad (1981–86), Chester A. Bond (1985–93), William Mellon (1986–), Curt A. Johnson (1993–96). The *Assistant Deans* have been: Kenneth A. Connors (1968–72), Phillip A. Hart (1972–73), W. Michael Dickson (1975–80), Daniel H. Rich (1975–80), Gordon L. Amidon (1976–80), Peter G. Welling (1976–80), Christine A. Sorkness (1986–90).

Besides the temporary administrative service by these faculty members, a full-time, permanent position was created at the end of the first century to assure professional management of the business affairs of the School. Tim J. Gossens became the first to hold this post as Assistant Dean for Administration (1983–93), then as Associate Dean (1993–).

Appendix 2

Pharmacy Faculty of the First Century

Compiled by Gregory J. Higby

FACULTY MEMBERS included on this historical roster held the rank of Instructor or above, had instructional duties between 1883 and 1983, and were listed as part of the pharmacy faculty in at least two primary sources contemporary to their time. Additionally, faculty employed after 1983 have been included for completeness. Each is listed under whichever of the following broad subject categories seemed to represent best his or her main expertise:

- pharmacy, pharmaceutics, pharmaceutical chemistry
- materia medica, pharmacognosy, pharmaceutical biochemistry
- pharmacology
- pharmacy practice, including hospital pharmacy
- pharmacy administration & jurisprudence; social & historical studies of pharmacy
- extension services, including UW–Milwaukee

Categorizing faculty—in the absence of formal departmentalization in the School—will be occasionally doubtful. For example, subject areas can change their character or overlap; instructors can evolve into new or restructured specialties over time. Any member of the teaching faculty with the rank of Instructor or above in a pharmacy-related field is listed, whether or not in a full-time appointment—including a few on the budget of the pharmacy department at $0 salary (e.g., an occasional "adjunct" professor, or a joint appointee salaried 100% on another department's budget). In a few instances where a faculty member's specialization was unclear, the listing has been placed under "pharmacy."Each listing consists of:

- Name and highest earned degree at the time of service (if degree is known).
- Highest academic rank held while at Wisconsin abbreviated as follows:

I	= Instructor	P	= Professor
L	= Lecturer	Cl	= Clinical
At P	= Assistant Professor	Sp	= Specialist
Ac P	= Associate Professor	Adj	= Adjunct

Note: Not listed are the occasional Visiting Professors and the part-time Clinical Instructors. Years on the School faculty include leaves of absence (e.g., for teaching or research elsewhere or military service). A gap within the period of service is signaled by a semi-colon. The table is arranged chronologically, by year of appointment in each category.

Pharmacy, Pharmaceutics, and Pharmaceutical Chemistry

Frederick B. Power, PhD
P 1883–92

Edward Kremers, PhD
I 1891–92 P 1892–1935

Louis Kahlenberg, PhD
I 1893–98[2]

Richard Fischer, PhD
I 1894–98 At P 1900–09

Oswald Schreiner, PhD
I 1897–1902

I. W. Brandel, MS
I 1902–05

Albert E. Kundert
I 1902–03

Frank Rabak, BS
I 1905–06

Andrew G. DuMez, BS
I 1907–09(?)

Nellie A. Wakeman, PhD
I 1913– At P 1928–46

Henry A. Langenhan, PhD
I 1913– At P 1922–23

Emery T. Motley
I 1923–24

Glenn L. Jenkins, PhD
I 1925–28

Bernard V. Christensen, MS
I 1925–28

Ralph W. Clark, PhD
I 1927–37

Arthur A. Harwood, PhD
I 1927–30

Arthur H. Uhl, PhD
I 1930–31 At P 1935–
Ac P 1937– P 1940–71

Karl J. Goldner, PhD
I 1937–40

Lloyd M. Parks, PhD
I 1937– At P 1940–
Ac 1945– P 1946–56

Louis W. Busse, PhD
I 1940– At P 1942–
Ac P 1945– P 1949–78

Melvin F. Dunker, PhD
At P 1942–45

Takeru Higuchi, PhD
At P 1947– Ac P 1950–
P 1954–67

Dale E. Wurster, PhD
I 1947 At P 1948–
Ac P 1952– P 1959–71

William O. Foye, PhD
At P 1949–55

Melvin W. Green, PhD
Ac P 1949–52

John A. Neptune, PhD
I 1952–55

August P. Lemberger, PhD
I 1953– At P 1955–
Ac P 1957– P 1963–69; 1980–91

Eino Nelson, PhD
I 1954–55

Edward E. Smissman, PhD
At P 1955– Ac P 1957–60

Hyman Mitchner, PhD[3]
I 1955– At P 1956–59

S. Morris Kupchan, PhD
At P 1957– Ac P 1959–
P 1961–69

William I. Higuchi, PhD
At P 1959–62

Stuart P. Eriksen, PhD
At P 1960– Ac P 1963–65

Jack R. Arndt, PhD
I 1961– Ac P 1976–77

Raymond W. Doskotch, PhD
At P 1961–63

Kenneth A. Connors, PhD
At P 1961– Ac P 1965–
P 1970–

George R. Flouret, PhD
At P 1962–64

John H. Perrin, PhD
At P 1962– Ac P 1968–73

John J. Windheuser, PhD
Ac P 1963–72

Phillip A. Hart, PhD
At P 1964– Ac P 1969–
P 1979–95

Virgil Lee, MS
I 1966–69

Joseph R. Robinson, PhD
At P 1966– Ac P 1970–
P 1974–

Pasupati Mukerjee, PhD
Ac P 1966–67 P 1967–94

Jens T. Carstensen, PhD
At P 1968– Ac P 1969–
P 1973–95

Darryle A. Weishaar, BS
Sp 1968–69

Robert A. Ellison, PhD
At P 1969–75

H. Perri Corrick-West, MS
I 1970–

Judith F. (Albers) Thompson, MS
I 1970–73; L 1987–
Cl At P 1991– Cl Ac P 1996–

Daniel H. Rich, PhD
At P 1970– Ac P 1975–
P 1981–

Robert B. Morin, PhD
Ac P 1971 73

Gordon L. Amidon, PhD
At P 1971– Ac P 1967–82

George Zografi, PhD
P 1972–

Peter G. Welling, PhD
At P 1972– Ac P 1975–
P 1978–84

John H. Young, PhD
At P 1973–75

Philip Mendel, BS
At Cl P 1978–87

C. Richard Hutchinson, PhD
At P 1975– Ac P 1977–
P 1983–

Lloyd Kennon, PhD
Ac P 1976–77

William R. Porter, PhD
At P 1978–84

Debra Fleisher, MS
L 1979–82

Brian C. Gunn, MS
L 1979–81

Margaret Lopachin, MS
L 1982–85

Ronald Burnette, PhD
At P 1982– Ac P 1988–

Timothy Heath, PhD
At P 1985– Ac P 1990–

James L. Wright, PhD
At P 1987–88
Adj At P 1990– Adj Ac P 1993–

Paul Hutson, PhD
At P 1988– Ac P 1991–

Guilherme Indig, PhD
At P 1995–

Materia Medica, Pharmacognosy, and Pharmaceutical Biochemistry

Frederick B. Power, PhD
P 1883–92

Lellen S. Cheney, PhD
I 1892– At P 1895–1903

Rodney H. True, PhD
At P 1895–99

Rollin H. Denniston, PhD[4]
I 1900–03 At P 1913–1918

William O. Richtmann, PhD
I 1898–99; 1901–02
At P 1919– Ac P 1927–
P 1935–47

S. R. Boyce
I 1900–03

Emerson R. Miller, MS[5]
At P 1913–1918

Joseph V. Swintosky, PhD
At P 1948– Ac P 1949–53

Joseph G. Cannon, PhD
At P 1956– Ac P 1960–62

Charles J. Sih, PhD
At P 1960– Ac P 1964–
P 1966–

David Perlman, PhD
P 1967–1980

Dexter B. Northrop, PhD
At P 1971– Ac P 1976–
P 1982–

Ulfert Hornemann, PhD
P 1981–

Margaret Claggett-Dame, PhD
At P 1989– Ac P 1995–

Catherine A. Royer, PhD
At P 1990–

Donald T. Witiak, PhD
P 1993–

Pharmacology

Kenneth F. Finger, PhD
Ac P 1962– P 1967–68

Robert N. Morris, PhD
At P 1966–71

Charles F. Ryan, Jr., PhD
At P 1969–73

Paul Bass, PhD
P 1970–

Carl K. Buckner, PhD
At P 1970– Ac P 1975–
P 1981–87

Thomas A. Rudy, PhD
At P 1971– Ac P 1976–
P 1982–

Gary C. Lage, PhD
Ac P 1973–79

Frederick W. Benz, PhD
At P 1973–79

Richard E. Peterson, PhD
At P 1975– Ac P 1979–
P 1984–

Ralph M. Albrecht, PhD
At P 1979– Ac P 1983–
P 1989–

William S. Mellon, PhD
At P 1979– Ac P 1984–

Robert Earhart, Jr., PhD
At P 1980–83

Molly Weiler, PhD
At P 1984–91

Warren Heideman, PhD
At P 1988– Ac P 1994–

Ellyn Wheeler-Clark, PhD
At P 1989–94

Pharmacy Practice including Hospital Pharmacy

Winston J. Durant, BS
At P 1960–71

David A. Zilz, MS
Sp 1968– At Cl P 1971–
Ac Cl P 1978– Cl P 1984–96

David Angaran, MS
Sp 1970– At Cl P 1973–76

Thomas S. Thielke, MS
Cl I 1970– At Cl P 1978–
Cl Ac P 1983– Cl P 1989–

Monte G. Cohon, PharmD
L 1971– At Cl P 1973–78

Peter P. Drozdowicz
Sp 1971–72

Pamela Palmer, BS
I 1973–74

Chester A. Bond, PharmD
Cl At P 1973– Cl Ac P 1979–
P 1986–96

Jean M. Nappi, PharmD
Cl At P 1977–80

Ronald L. Sorkness, PhD
Cl At P 1977– Cl Ac P 1981–
Ac P 1994–

Curtis A. Johnson, PharmD
Cl At P 1978– Ac P 1981–
P 1987–

Christine A. (Sczupak) Sorkness, PharmD
Cl At P 1979– Cl Ac P 1981–
P 1987–

Steven Bauwens, MS
Cl At P 1980– Cl Ac P 1986–
Ac P 1987–88

Arthur Schuna, MS
Cl At P 1980– Cl Ac P 1983–93
Cl P 1993–

William Craig, MD
Ac P 1980–83 P 1983–

Pamela Ploetz, BS
Cl At P 1981–

Cynthia Raehl, PharmD
Cl At P 1981– Cl Ac P 1986–
P 1992–96

Larry E. Boh, MS
Cl At P 1982– At P 1987–
Ac P 1988– P 1994–

Linda S. Tyler
Cl At P 1981–84

Wendy Weingart
Cl At P 1982–84

Michael Pitterle, MS
Cl At P 1985– At P 1987–
Ac P 1991–

Steven C. Ebert, PharmD
Cl At P 1985– At P 1987–90

Paul Pisarzewicz
Cl At P 1988–89

Richard Hammes
Cl At P 1988–

Kathryn Grant
Cl At P 1988–95

Roberta Carrier, PharmD
Cl At P 1988–92

Marilyn Bufton
Cl At P 1989–

Donald Michalski
Cl At P 1990–

William Reiss, PharmD
At P 1991–93

Timothy Hoon, PharmD
At P 1991–

Barry Gidal, PharmD
At P 1991– Ac P 1996–

Ann Nutt
Cl At P 1993–94

Akiko Hoon
Cl At P 1993–

Shelly Gray, PharmD
At P 1992–95

Allan T. Mailloux, PharmD
At P 1993–97

Karen MacKenzie
Adj At P 1989–

Cynthia M. Horton, PharmD
At P 1993–

Connie Kraus, PharmD
Cl At P 1993–

Pharmacy Administration and Jurisprudence; Social and Historical Studies of Pharmacy

George Urdang, Dr rer nat
P 1947–52

William S. Apple, PhD[6]
I 1951– At P 1954–
Ac P 1957–58

Glenn A. Sonnedecker, PhD
At P 1952– Ac P 1956–
P 1960–86

Ernst W. Stieb, PhD
I 1958– At P 1959–
Ac P 1964–67

Robert W. Hammel, PhD
At P 1958– Ac P 1962–
P 1968–90

Richard A. Ohvall, PhD
At P 1964– Ac P 1968–1971

John L. Parascandola, PhD
At P 1969– Ac P 1973–
P 1980–83

Kenneth W. Kirk, PhD
At P 1972–75

W. Michael Dickson, PhD
At P 1974– Ac P 1979–80

Bonnie L. Svarstad, PhD
At P 1975– Ac P 1980–
P 1986–

Joseph Wiederholt, PhD
At P 1981– Ac P 1988–

David Kreling, PhD
At P 1984– Ac P 1990–

Jeanine Mount, PhD
At P 1985– Ac P 1992–

John Scarborough, PhD
P 1985–

Thomas McGregor, BS
Adj At P 1986–

Gregory J. Higby, PhD
Adj At P 1986– Adj Ac P 1994–

Betty Chewning, PhD
Adj Ac P 1988– At P 1993–

Extension and UW-Milwaukee

Eunice Bonow Bardell, PhD
Ac P 1952–72

Charles H. Barnstein, PhD
Ac P 1963–70

William L. Blockstein, PhD
Ac P 1964– P 1967–91

Melvin H. Weinswig, PhD
P 1969–

Dindayal Patel, PhD
At P 1971–72

Alan L. Hanson, PhD[8]
Cl I 1973– At P 1979–
Ac P 1983– P 1989–

James DeMuth, PhD
At P 1974– Ac P 1979–
P 1984–

Michael Mergener, PhD
At P 1980–83

Editor's Note: In addition, academic staff have played an important and increasing instructional role in the School of Pharmacy, as in other departments of the University. While it is not feasible to identify all who have thus served the School since the founding, their essential role over the years is illustrated by the following list of Academic Staff who had served at least a decade as the School embarked on its second century: H. Perri Corrick-West (1970–); Gary G. Girdaukas (1972–); Tim J. Gossens, (1983–); Richard Krumbiegel (1971–96); Laurence E. Mindel (1978–); Pamela A. Palmer (1972–77, 1983–92, 1995–).

Pharmacy Library: A full-time Librarian has been on duty in the School only since the F. B. Power Pharmaceutical Library was established in 1950 as an official branch of the University Library. Since then the Librarians have been James Jones, Elsa Reich, and Dolores Nemec.

Notes

1. To determine who served on the pharmacy-related teaching faculty of the School, the following sources were utilized: University of Wisconsin Course in Pharmacy Announcement (1883–90); University of Wisconsin Catalog(ue) (1887–1929) and University of Wisconsin Announcement of Courses (1929–65); University of Wisconsin (–Madison) Directory [staff] (1940–96); Bulletin of the University of Wisconsin School of Pharmacy (1959–79); and the University of Wisconsin [System] Budget (Staff Detail). The latter was utilized as final authority in instances of doubtful status, except in the decade 1883–93, for which no budget books are in the University of Wisconsin–Madison Archives. For those years, printed course descriptions were examined, and only those faculty members whose courses were of a specifically pharmaceutical nature are included in the list.
2. Kahlenberg continued on at Wisconsin in the Chemistry Department from 1898 to 1929: At P 1898- P 1900–1929.
3. Mitchner started as an Instructor in the second semester of the 1955–56 school year.

4. Denniston was At P in the Botany Department from 1907–19. In addition, he was Curator of the Drug Cabinet from 1900 to 1919.
5. Miller was a plant chemist from the U.S. Department of Agriculture working at the Pharmaceutical Experiment Station.
6. Also served as Coordinator of Pharmacy Extension Services.
7. Only faculty members of Extension Services in Pharmacy who were listed in the School of Pharmacy budget are included in this section. Faculty not listed in the School budget have included W. Allen Daniels, Richard S. Strommen, James E. DeMuth, and Michael A. Mergener.
8. Hanson was an Instructor in the pharmaceutical dispensing course from 1973 to 1978.

APPENDIX 3

What Students Studied

THE REQUIRED and optional curricula below are transcribed verbatim from the indicated editions of the University's Catalogue or the Announcement of Courses, which varied in the style and detail of presentation. These lists of courses do not show, of course, the interim fine-tuning of each curriculum as it evolved over the years, nor the various pharmaceutical electives.

The Two-Year Curriculum, Required (as of the 1906–07 Catalogue)

Leading to the diploma of Graduate in Pharmacy (Ph.G.)

Note: For a transcription of the curriculum as it first appeared in the 1883–84 *Catalogue*, see Chapter I, p. 27. The curriculum is shown below, in more detail as it had matured over a period of twenty-three years.

First Year, First Semester

Chemistry 3* General chemistry: The laboratory work accompanying this course is especially designed for pharmacy students. Eight-fifths credit. Assoc. Prof. Lenher and Mr. Sievers.

Biology 1. General Biology: Introductory to both botany and zoology, and required as preliminary to all work in either department. Two recitations, or lectures, and eight hours laboratory work a week. Prof. Harper, Prof. Allen, and assistants.

Botany 25. The Collection and Commerce of Crude Drugs. Laboratory and field work supplemented by lectures and recitations. One-fifth. Dr. Denniston.

Pharmacy I. Laboratory Technique. The principles and practice of pharmaceutical operations, such as comminution, expression, decantation, filtration, maceration, percolation, diffusion, dialysis, crystallization and precipitation. Three-fifths. W., F., at 11. Miss Gage.

First Year, Second Semester

Chemistry 3. General Chemistry continued as a three-fifths study.

Chemistry 10. Qualitative Analysis. First half of semester, daily. Prof. Daniels and Mr. Sievers.

Chemistry 15. Quantitative Analysis. Second half of semester, daily. Prof. Daniels and Mr. Sievers.

---

*The figures refer to the numbers of the courses as given in the statements under Departments of Instruction.

Chemistry 20b. Organic Chemistry for Pharmacy students. Two-fifths course. Recitations and laboratory work. Dr. Koelker and Mr. Sievers.

Botany 20. Morphology and Classification of the Flowering Plants. An elementary course designed primarily for students in Pharmacy. The life histories and ecology of seed plants, with a comparative study of the structure of the principal families and the identification of common species. Field work will be an important feature. Excursions on Saturdays. M., T., W., Th., F., 8 to 10. Dr. Olive and Mr. Reed.

Pharmacy 1. Laboratory Technique. Continuation, work of the first semester. (See above.)

Second Year, First Semester

Chemistry 6. Advanced Inorganic Chemistry. Lectures and recitations, Tu., Th., F., at 10: laboratory work daily. Prof. Kremers and Mr. Schulz.

Chemistry 40. Plant Chemistry. As a three-fifths study supplementary to pharmacognosy. Recitation, Mon., at 10; two laboratory periods. Professor Kremers and Miss Gage.

Botany 5. Vegetable Histology. A systematic study of the tissues of the phanerogams and ferns. Use of reagents and stains, section cutting and mounting. Dr. Denniston and Mr. Lutman.

Botany 22. Pharmacognosy. This course presents to the student the main facts of the natural history of drugs, and the plants producing them. Twice a week throughout the senior year. Dr. Denniston.

Pharmacy 2. Pharmaceutical Technology. The study and manufacture of galenical and other preparations: waters, tinctures, fluid extracts, spirits, oleoresins, etc.; also of pills, suppositories, ointments, plasters, etc. lectures and recitations, Tu., Th., at 11; three laboratory periods. Assistant Professor Fischer and Mr. Du Mez.

Second Year, Second Semester

Chemistry 27. Advanced Organic Chemistry. Lectures and recitations, Tu., Th., F., at 10; laboratory work daily. Professor Kremers and Mr. Schulz.

Chemistry 40. Plant Chemistry. Continued from first semester. Prof. Kremers and Miss Gage.

Chemistry 45. Alkaloidal Assay. One-fifth credit. Assist. Prof. Fischer and Mr. Du Mez.

Botany 21. Microscopical Examination of Drugs and Food Products. The object of this course is to study and illustrate the methods of identifying powdered drugs and food products and detecting adulterations. Three-fifths credit. Dr. Denniston.

Botany 22. Pharmacognosy. Continuation of first semester's work. Dr. Denniston.

Pharmacy 3. Prescription Practice. The study of the prescription; practice in the compounding of physicians' prescriptions; also the study of physical, chemical and therapeutical incompatibilities. Lectures and recitations, Tu., Th., at 11; two laboratory periods. Assist. Prof. Fischer and Mr. Du Mez.

The Initial Three-Year Curriculum, Optional (as of the 1896–97 Catalogue)

Leading to the diploma of Graduate in Pharmacy (Ph.G.)

Sophomore Year

Chemistry, 1; Pharmaceutical Botany, 1 or Biology, 1; Pharmaceutical Technique, 1; Electives.

Junior Year

Chemistry, 5; Pharmaceutical Chemistry, 1 and 2; Pharmaceutical Botany, 2, 3 and 4; Pharmaceutical Technique; Pharmacognosy, 1; Practical Pharmacy, 3; Electives.

Senior Year

Pharmacognosy, 1 and 2; Practical Pharmacy, 1 and 2; Thesis; Electives.

> *The availability of this third curricular option was announced in the Catalogue for 1894–95, but the detail of coursework was not published until 1896–97, as above.*—The Editor

The Second Three-Year Curriculum, Required (as of 1925–26 Catalogue)

Leading to the diploma of Graduate in Pharmacy (Ph.G.)

First Year

First Semester	Credits	Second Semester	Credits
Engl. 1a-Freshman Composition	3	Engl. 1b-Freshman Composition	3
Chem. 1a-General Chemistry	5	Chem. 1b-Qualitative Analysis	5
Bot. 1-General Botany	5	Chem. 15-Quantitative Analysis	2
Pharm. 1-Pharmaceut. Technique	3	Bot. 130-Seed Plants	3
Physical Education or		Pharm. 1-Pharmaceut. Technique	3
Military Science	*0*	Physical Education or Military Science	*0*
	16		16

Second Year

First Semester	Credits	Second Semester	Credits
Chem. 20-Organic Chemistry	4	Chem. 27-Pharmaceutical Chem.	5
Chem. 26-Pharmaceutical Chem.	5	Bot. 111-Microscopic Examination	3
Bot. 100-Plant Histology	3	Pharm. 20-Elementary Prescription	
Practice	2		
Pharm. 20-Elem. Prescr. Practice	2	Pharmacog. 10-Sources of Drugs	1
Pharmacog. 10-Sources of Drugs	1	Pharm. 40-Drug Store Practice	1
Pharm. 40-Drug Store Practice	1	Electives	4
Physical Ed. or Military Science	0	Physical Ed. or Military Science	0
	16		16

Third Year

First Semester	Credits	Second Semester	Credits
Pharm. 30-Pharmaceutical Tech.	4	Pharm. 30-Pharmaceutical Tech.	4
Pharm. 121-Advanced Prescription		Pharm. 121-Advanced Prescription	
Practice	1	Practice	1
Pharmacog. 20-Crude Drugs	3	Pharmacog. 20-Crude Drugs	3
Chem. 40-Plant Chemistry	3	Chem. 40-Plant Chemistry	3
Pharm. 50-History of Pharmacy	1	Chem. 45-Alkaloid Assay	1
Pharm. 100-Thesis	2	Pharm. 50-History of Pharmacy	1
Electives	2	Pharm. 100-Thesis	2
		Electives	4
	16		16 [sic]

Eight of the ten elective credits must be taken outside of the Departments of Pharmacy, Chemistry, and Botany.

The Initial Four-Year Curriculum, Optional (1892–93 Catalogue)

Leading to the degree of Bachelor of Science (Pharmacy)

Freshman Year: Biology, 1; German, 9; Mathematics, 1,2,3; English, 2; Hygiene, 1, military drill, gymnastics, 3 hours weekly.

Sophomore Year: French, 3; Chemistry, 1,2,3; Physics, 2; English, 3; military drill, gymnastics, 3 hours weekly.

Junior and Senior Years: Pharmaceutical chemistry and botany must be taken for two years. If chemistry is elected as major study, botany must be taken as assigned minor, or vice versa. The elective minor study can be made up of a series of courses or of a single continuous course, and must be at least equivalent to a full study throughout the last two years of the course.

With regard to synoptical lectures and rules of the Group System, compare pages 53–55 [of the catalog].

The Four-Year Curriculum, Required (1931–32 Catalogue)

Leading to the degree of Bachelor of Science (Pharmacy)

The First Two Years

	Credits
English 1-Freshman composition	6
Biology 1-General Biology (including elementary botany	10
Chemistry 1-General chemistry and qualitative analysis	10
Physics 1 or 31-General physics	10
Pharmacy 1-Orientation in pharmacy	6
Pharmacy 20-Elementary prescription practice	4
French-Reading knowledge	0–14
German-Reading knowledge	14–0
Physical activity requirement (four semesters)	0
	60

The Last Two Years

	Credits
Botany 110, 111-Pharmaceutical botany	6
Pharm. Chem. 26, 27-Organic and inorganic pharmaceutical chemistry	10
Pharm. Chem. 45-Pharmaceutical assaying	4
Pharm. Chem. 40-Plant chemistry	6
Pharmacognosy 10-Crude vegetable and animal drugs	2
Pharmacognosy 120-Natural history of drugs	6
Pharmacy 30-Pharmaceutical technology	5
Pharmacy 121-Advanced prescription practice	2
Pharmacy 51-Drug store practice	2
Pharmacy 50-History of pharmacy	2
Thesis	4
Electives	11
	60

Final Version, Four-Year Curriculum, Required (1956–58 Catalog)

Leading to the degree of Bachelor of Science (Pharmacy)

First Semester	Credits	Second Semester	Credits
Freshman Year			
English 1a-Freshman English	3	English 1b-Freshman English	3
Chemistry 1a-General chemistry	5	Chemistry 1b-General chemistry	5
Mathematics or Language	4	Mathematics or Language	4
Botany 17-Survey	3	Zoology 17-Survey	3
Pharmacy 1a-Orientation	1	Pharmacy 1b-Orientation	1
Physical Education	0	Physical Education	0
Military Training or Band	0	Military Training or Band	0
	16		16
Sophomore Year			
Pharm. Chem. 24a	3	Pharm. Chem. 24b	3
Pharm. Chem. 25a	1	Pharm. Chem. 25b	1
Pharmacy 3	2	Pharmacy 4	4
Physics 65	3	Physics 65	3
Bacteriology 1	4	Electives	5–6
Electives	3–4	Physical Education (women only)	0
Physical Education (women only)	0	Military Training	0
Military Training	0		
	16–17		16–17
Junior Year			
Pharm. Chem. 126	3	Pharm. Chem. 127	4
Pharm. Chem. 145	4	Pharmacognosy 120b	3
Pharmacy 128	2	Physiology 103	5
Pharmacy 129	2	Electives	4–5
Pharmacognosy 120a	3		
Electives	2–3		
	16–17		16–17
Senior Year			
Pharmacy 134	2	Pharm. Chem. 140b	4
Pharmacy 135	2	Pharm. Chem. 146	2
Pharm. Chem. 140a	4	Pharmacy 150	2
Pharmacy 142	4	Pharmacy 151	2
Pharmacy 158	3	*Pharmacy 100	0–2
*Pharmacy 100	0–2	Electives	6–5
Electives	2–0		
	17	1	6–17

*Students who have a grade-point average of 2.5 or better may elect 4 credits of Thesis

The Initial Five-Year Curriculum, Required (1959–61 Catalogue)

Leading to the Degree of Bachelor of Science (Pharmacy)

The specific requirements for admission to the School of Pharmacy which should be met by the end of the sophomore year are:

	Credits
English Composition	6
Chemistry	16
General Inorganic and Qualitative Analysis	8
Organic	8
Mathematics	8
General Physics	6
Biological Science (Zoology and Botany)	6
Economics	3
Electives	
To a Total of	60

Pharmacy-First Year

Pharmacy 150	4	Pharmacy 154	3
Pharmacy 153	3	Pharm. Chem. 121	5
Pharm. Chem. 102	2	Microbiology	5
Pharm. Chem. 105	4	Elective	3
Elective	3		
	16		16

Pharmacy-Second Year

Physiology 103	5	Pharmacology 142	5
Pharmacy 162	3	Pharm. Chem. 106	3
Pharm. Chem. 123	4	Pharmacy 155	2
Pharmacognosy 130	4	Pharmacy 156	2
		Pharmacognosy 131	4
	16		16

Pharmacy-Third Year

Pharmacy 165	2	Pharmacy 167	2
Pharmacy 166	2	Pharmacy 168	3
Pharmacognosy 133	2	Pharm. Admin. 117	2
Pharmacology 143	2	Pharmacy 101	1
Technical Electives*	8	Technical Electives*	8
	16		16

*Technical Electives must be selected in an integrated program of study from among the options given below:

First Semester	[Technical Electives] Credits	Second Semester	Credits
Professional Pharmacy			
Pharm. Admin. 108a	3	Pharm. Admin. 118	3
Pharm. Admin. 112	3	Pharmacy 160	1
Elective	2	Elective	4
	8		8
Hospital Pharmacy			
Pharmacy 158	3	Pharmacy 171	3
Pharmacy 175	2	Hosp. Pharm. Admin. 115	3
Elective	3	Elective	2
	8		8
Industrial Pharmacy			
Pharmacy 158	3	Pharmacy 171	3
Pharmacy 175	2	Pharmacy 178	3
Elective	3	Elective	2
	8		8

Pregraduate Study

Basic science deficiencies [to be remedied] depending upon student's academic background and selected major area of study.

A Modified Five-Year Curriculum, Required (1977–79 Catalogue)

Leading to the degree of Bachelor of Science (Pharmacy)

[*Editor's Note*: Striking alterations to the five-year curriculum occurred during the 1970s to adapt to the concept of "clinical pharmacy" as a mode of practice. The flow chart on the next page was published in 1977 to clarify the logical structure of the curriculum, supplementing curriculum tables in the Announcement of Courses (Bull. Univ. Wis, 1977–1979, No. 9). The sequence of a student's three professional years in the School begins at the bottom, separated by horizontal lines. The two pre-pharmacy years were not altered in the subjects required (since 1959); but the *level* of knowledge required increased somewhat in mathematics, physics, chemistry, and economics.]

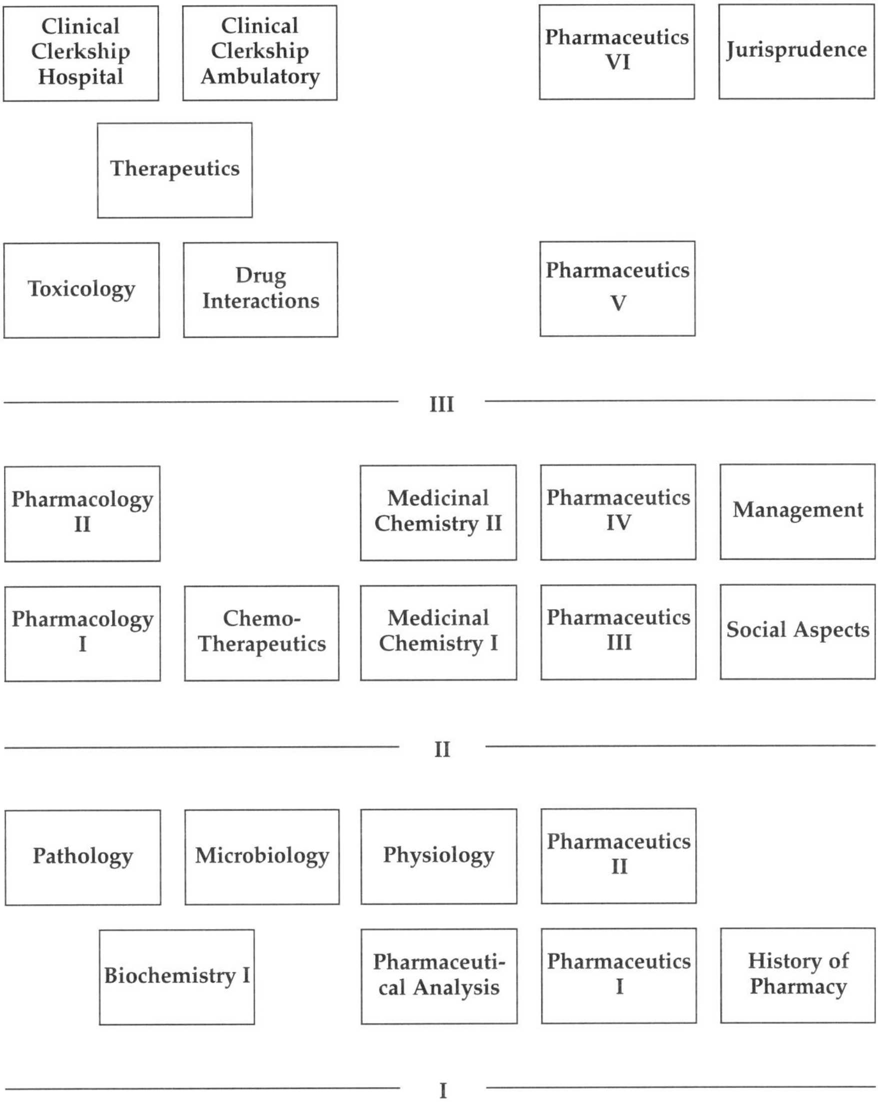
Clinical Clerkship Hospital
Clinical Clerkship Ambulatory
Pharmaceutics VI
Jurisprudence
Therapeutics
Toxicology
Drug Interactions
Pharmaceutics V
III
Pharmacology II
Medicinal Chemistry II
Pharmaceutics IV
Management
Pharmacology I
Chemo-Therapeutics
Medicinal Chemistry I
Pharmaceutics III
Social Aspects
II
Pathology
Microbiology
Physiology
Pharmaceutics II
Biochemistry I
Pharmaceutical Analysis
Pharmaceutics I
History of Pharmacy
I

APPENDIX 4

The Students

TABLES OF ENROLLMENTS AND DEGREES COMPILED BY GREGORY J. HIGBY.
TABLES OF AWARDS COMPILED BY SANDRA C. GOSSENS.

• Enrollments • Degrees conferred • Awards for academic excellence

Appendix 4a: Undergraduate Pharmacy Enrollment, 1883–1983

	2-Yr. Ph.G.			3-Yr. Ph.G.			B.S. Pharm.			
	Total	Women	Out-of-State	Total	Women	Out-of-State	Total	Women	Out-of-State	All-U.W.†
1883–84	27	0	0							388
1884–85	41	5	1							387
1885–86	40	2	5							421
1886–87	47	1	0							505
1887–88	37	3	2							637
1888–89	49	2	1							722
1889–90	35	1	3							789
1890–91	56	2	1							966
1891–92	63	3	4							1092
1892–93	62	2	3				2	0	0	1287
1893–94	37	2	0				4	0	0	1279
1894–95	17	1	1	13	2	0	8	2	1	1520
1895–96	16	0	0	17	5	1	13	2	2	1598
1896–97	20	1	0	29	4	3	11	2	1	1650
1897–98	16	0	0	34	3	1	9	2	0	1767
1898–99	18	2	0	29	3	5	6	1	0	1923
1899–00	19	4	2	22	1	3	7	1	2	2422
1900–01	17	1	1	20	2	6	7	1	0	2619

continued

	2-Yr. Ph.G.			3-Yr. Ph.G.			B.S. Pharm.			
	Total	Women	Out-of-State	Total	Women	Out-of-State	Total	Women	Out-of-State	All-U.W.
1901–02	14	1	1	13	1	0	5	2	0	2777
1902–03	20	0	1	8	0	2	5	0	0	2870
1903–04	28	1	2				7	1	1	3151
1904–05	26	0	2				6	1	1	3342
1905–06	26	1	3				5	0	0	3571
1906–07	27	1	3				8	2	0	3659
1907–08	24	2	0				8	2	1	4013
1908–09	32	1	0				8	0	0	
1909–10	36	1	1				4	0	0	4947
1910–11	36	1	1	4	0	0	6	0	0	5538
1911–12	26	2	4				12	0	0	5748
1912–13	27	3	5				14	0	1	5970
1913–14	24	1	1				16	0	1	6765
1914–15	21	4	1				10	1	2	7596
1915–16	27	5	1				9	0	0	7624
1916–17	41	7	4				8	2	0	8121
1917–18	26	5	5				9	2	1	6367
1918–19	19	1	3				10	1	2	6978
1919–20	74	4	4				19	2	4	7294
1920–21	68	8	4				21	5	6	7471
1921–22	56	4	7				40	7	9	7756
1922–23	53	1	5				37	6	8	8044
1923–24	60	1	4				44	6	11	8076
1924–25	59	1	0				51	12	*	8351

continued

†All-University enrollment figures include undergraduate students, graduate students, professional students, special students, and part-time students—although data from early years might have been less inclusive occasionally.

*The hometown of each student was no longer listed after the UW *Catalogue* of 1923–24.

	2-Yr. Ph.G.			3-Yr. Ph.G.			B.S. Pharm.			
	Total	**Women**	**Out-of-State**	**Total**	**Women**	**Out-of-State**	**Total**	**Women**	**Out-of-State**	**All-U.W.**
1925–26				67	4	*	57	14		8331
1926–27				46	?		54	?		8836
1927–28				54	8		63	7		9672
1928–29				50	5		40	4		9746
1929–30				61	6		36	3		10077
1930–31				59	3		17	3		10001
1931–32				47	1		34	4		9355
1932–33				31	0		49	6		8423
1933–34				14	0		56	9		7957
1934–35				3	0		85	14		8657

continued

	B.S. Pharm.		
	Total Students	Women	All-U.W.
1935–36	112	23	9617
1936–37	113	16	10679
1937–38	108	17	11552
1938–39	117	14	12134
1939–40	134	14	11949
1940–41	162	14	12012
1941–42	161	14	11133
1942–43	117	15	9466
1943–44	55	28	5666 civilians
1944–45	46	25	6711 civilians
1945–46	92	51	13543 civilians
1946–47	360	43?	19882
1947–48	426	55	19959
1948–49	403	46	19918
1949–50	411	39	19184
1950–51	296	29	17197
1951–52	268	33	15082
1952–53	260	30	14868
1953–54	232	27	14725
1954–55	198	18	15377
1955–56	225	25	16553
1956–57	257	38	17576
1957–58	215	34	18007
1958–59	221	32	18825
1959–60	217	31	18953
1960–61	274	40	20314
1961–62	206	26	21574
1962–63	213	30	23378

continued

	B.S. Pharm.		
	Total Students	Women	All-U.W.
1963–64	178	22	25924
1964–65	262	33	28068
1965–66	280	34	31100
1966–67	341	50	33006
1967–68	397	72	33000
1968–69	460	94	34670
1969–70	437	86	35616
1970–71	447	73	34445
1971–72	474	79	33943
1972–73	502	103	37687
1973–74	494	115	38315
1974–75	512	130	36915
1975–76	525	161	38545
1976–77	527	175	37924
1977–78	533	192	38947
1978–79	529	190	39430
1979–80	506	204	40129
1980–81	451	190	41242
1981–82	407	186	41691
1982–83	349	174	42230

Pharmacy enrollment figures obtained from the following sources:

University of Wisconsin(-Madison) Catalogues and School of Pharmacy Bulletins (1883–1943); University telephone directories (women) and School of Pharmacy records, Kremers Reference Files (men) (1943–46); "First-Semester Enrollment Figures," U.W. Archives 1947–52; "Undergraduate Enrollment," document from U.W. Registrar's Office (1952–58, 1978–81); annual enrollment figures from *Am J Pharm Ed* (1959–78). Total U.W. enrollment figures from: University Catalogues (1883–1967 *except* 1940–41, 1943–46; "University of Wisconsin Enrollments (Madison Campus)," document from "Enrollment" folder in U.W. Archives, vertical subject file 1940–41, 1943–46; *Opening Fall Enrollment in Higher Education* (1967–76); *Collegiate Enrollment in the United States* (1976–1981).

Appendix 4b: Graduate Students in the School of Pharmacy

Year	Enrollment	Year	Enrollment
1950	46	1973	78
1951	47	1974	79
1952	46	1975	81
1953	50	1976	92
1954	50	1977	93
1955	55	1978	78
1956	64	1979	76
1957	72	1980	84
1958	73	1981	93
1959	79	1982	91
1960	67	1983	92
1961	83	1984	85
1962	74	1986	72
1963	89	1987	71
1964	95	1988	75
1965	95	1989	77
1966	95	1990	75
1967	84	1991	65
1968	72	1992	67
1969	67	1993	68
1970	60	1994	55
1971	64	1995	62
1972	65		

Total enrollment in the fall semester of each academic year tabulated. While enrollments for 1893–1949 were not accessible for inclusion in the present table, the number of degrees conferred annually suggests that having a total enrollment of more than a dozen graduate students before the 1940s was exceptional.

Appendix 4c: Degrees Conferred in Pharmacy Programs, 1883–1983

	Diplomas PhG Program		Degrees BS Pharmacy		Total Pharm.	% Women	Graduate Degrees
	Total	Women	Total	Women			Total conferred* and, in paren, number of women
1883–1884	3						
1884–1885	8						
1885–1886	10						
1886–1887	14						
1887–1888	9						
1888–1889	16						
1889–1890	8						
1890–1891	16						
1891–1892	14	2				14	
1892–1893	14						
1893–1894	12						1 Ph M
1894–1895	8	1	1		9	11	
1895–1896	7	1	3		10	10	
1896–1897	6		3		9	0	
1897–1898	10	1	5	2	15	20	
1898–1899	14	3?	2		16	19	1 MS (Chem)
1899–1900	11	1	1		12	8	1 MS (1)
1900–1901	15	1	4		19	5	
1901–1902	6		2	2	8	25	1 MS, 1 MPh, PhD (Chem)
1902–1903	9		2		11	0	
1903–1904	8		1		9	0	1 MS (Chem)
1904–1905	10		2	1	12	8	1 MA (1) (Chem)
1905–1906	10	1	1		11	9	1 PhD (?)
1906–1907	11		2		13	0	1 MPh
1907–1908	7	1	3	2	10	30	
1908–1909	4		4		8	0	

continued

	Diplomas PhG Program		Degrees, BS Pharmacy		Total Pharm.	% Women	Graduate Degrees
	Total	Women	Total	Women			Total conferred* and, in paren, number of women
1909–1910	11		3		14	0	2 MS (1) (Chem)
1910–1911	16				16	0	1 MS (Chem)
1911–1912	13	1	2		15	7	1 MA (Chem)
1912–1913	7	1	4		11	9	1 PhD (Bot & Chem) (1)
1913–1914	7		5		12	0	
1914–1915	8	1	3		11	9	1 MS, 1 PhD (Chem)
1915–1916	8		2		10	0	1 MS, 2 PhD (?)
1916–1917	7	2			7	29	1 PhD (DuMez)
1917–1918	14		3		17	0	1 PhD
1918–1919	4		3	1	7	14	1 MS, 1 PhD
1919–1920	14		3		17	0	2 PhD
1920–1921	19	2	3		22	9	1 PhD (Chem)
1921–1922	16	2	8	1	24	13	2 MS, 1 PhD
1922–1923	17		8	2	25	8	3 MS
1923–1924	12	1?	11		23	4	2 MS
1924–1925	10		8	3	18	17	4 MS (1), 1 PhD
1925–1926	12		12	1	24	4	3 MS, 5 PhD
1926–1927	15		9	3	24	13	5 MS, 1 PhD
1927–1928	6	1	11	2	17	18	1 MS, 3 PhD
1928–1929	6	2	9		15	13	5 MS, 2 PhD
1929–1930	13	2?	15	1	28	11	2 MS, 3 PhD
1930–1931	21	1	2		23	4	3 MS, 4 PhD
1931–1932	10		5		15	0	3 MS, 2 PhD
1932–1933	16	1	12	2	28	11	1 MS (1), 5 PhD (1)
1933–1934	9		8	1	17	6	3 MS (2), 4 PhD
1934–1935	6		7	3	13	23	3 PhD
1935–1936			21	2?	21	10	2 MS, 3 PhD (2)
1936–1937			30	8		27	1 MS, 1 PhD

continued

	Diplomas PhG Program		Degrees, BS Pharmacy		Total Pharm.	% Women	Graduate Degrees
	Total	Women	Total	Women			Total conferred* and, in paren, number of women
1937–1938			29	6		21	1 MS, 5 PhD (1)
1938–1939			20	4		20	1 MS
Total number women to 1940 = 76							
1939–1940	1		19	3	20	15	2 MS, 4 PhD
1940–1941			26	3		12	5 PhD
1941–1942			27	3		11	1 PhD
1942–1943			34	2		6	5 PhD
1943–1944			13	4		31	None
1944–1945			3	1		33	3 MS, (1)
1945–1946			8	4		50	None
1946–1947			29	4		14	3 MS, 2 PhD
1947–1948			65	6		9	3 MS, 1 PhD
1948–1949			85	12		14	3 MS (1), 5 PhD
1949–1950			105	7		7	9 MS (4), 4 PhD
1950–1951			103	9		9	7 MS, 1 PhD
1951–1952			88	4		5	16 MS (2?), 11 PhD (3)
1952–1953			92	16		17	11 MS (1), 1 PhD
1953–1954			92	9		10	9 MS (1), 15 PhD (1)
1954–1955			71	9		13	5 MS, 8 PhD
1955–1956			61	6		10	9 MS (1), 9 PhD
1956–1957			76	9		12	6 MS (1), 6 PhD
1957–1958			95	13		14	8 MS (?), 12 PhD
1958–1959			77	11		14	6 MS, 16 PhD
1959–1960			51	7		14	9 MS, 11 PhD
1960–1961			64	7		11	14 MS (2?), 16 PhD (1?)
1961–1962			76	8		11	11 MS (1?), 7 PhD (1?)
1962–1963			95	12		13	14 MS, 12 PhD
1963–1964			24	5		21	12 MS (1), 14 PhD (1)

continued

	Diplomas PhG Program		Degrees, BS Pharmacy		Total Pharm.	% Women	Graduate Degrees
	Total	Women	Total	Women			Total conferred* and, in paren, number of women
1964–1965			72	9		13	19 MS (3), 13 PhD (2)
1965–1966			78	9		12	13 MS, 13 PhD
1966–1967			96	15		16	24 MS (4), 17 PhD (1)
1967–1968			79	10		13	20 MS (1), 10 PhD
1968–1969			129	23		18	24 MS (4), 17 PhD (2)
1969–1970			138	33		24	11 MS (2), 14 PhD (1)
1970–1971			138	22		16	14 MS (4), 9 PhD
1971–1972			114	23		20	9 MS (1), 8 PhD
1972–1973			149	29		19	13 MS (4), 7 PhD (1)
1973–1974			154	28		18	3 MS, 14 PhD (1)
1974–1975			150	30		20	17 MS (2), 7 PhD
1975–1976			158	45		28	14 MS (1), 4 PhD (1)
1976–1977			164	51		31	17 MS (1), 7 PhD
1977–1978			153	58		38	17 MS (4), 8 PhD
1978–1979			169	51		30	14 MS (4), 7 PhD
1979–1980			163	68		42	14 MS (5), 16 PhD (3)
1980–1981			167	65		39	11 MS (2), 6 PhD (1)
1981–1982			144	58		40	14 MS (6), 12 PhD (4)
1982–1983			115	54		47	13 MS (4), 7 PhD (1)

Sources:

Undergraduate: University of Wisconsin Catalogue (1884–1924); loose-leaf list of graduates and theses (1884–1964) in F.B. Power Pharmaceutical Library and 4310 Chamberlin Hall (untitled) (1925–1964); document entitled "Degrees Conferred" from University of Wisconsin Office of the Registrar (1964–1980).

Graduate: Loose-leaf list (above) (1884–1964); document "Degrees Conferred" (above)(1964–1980).

---

* Several graduate students earned a Ph.D. under the supervision of Edward Kremers before 1917, but the degree was granted through the Chemistry Department because of administrative requirements at the time. For more information on the granting of these early Ph.D.s, see Ernst W. Stieb's unpublished paper in the KRF, C31(a)I: Wisc. Similarly, 21 students of pharmacy administration earned an M.B.A. through a collaborative program with the School of Commerce, 1951 through 1962, before Pharmacy's program was authorized to offer a graduate major. Hence, the degrees of these students are not included in the table.

Appendix 4d: Graduate Degrees Conferred for Work in the School

COMPILED BY KENNETH A. CONNORS

Year	M.A.	M.S.	M.B.A.	Ph.D.
1893		1		
1899		1		
1900		1		
1902		1		1
1904	1			
1905	1			
1906	1			1
1910	1	2		
1911		1		
1912	1			
1913				1
1915		1		1
1916		1		2
1917				1
1918	1	1		2
1919		1		1
1920				2
1921				1
1922		2		1
1923		3		
1924		2		
1925		4		1
1926		3		6
1927		5		1
1928	1	1		3
1929		5		2
1930		2		3
1931		3		4
1932		3		2
1933		1		5
1934		3		4
1935				3
1936	1	2		3
1937				1
1938		1		5

Year	M.A.	M.S.	M.B.A.	Ph.D.
1939		1		
1940		1		4
1941				5
1942				1
1943				5
1945		3		
1947		3		2
1948		3		1
1949		3		5
1950		9		4
1951		8	1	1
1952		16		10
1953		11		1
1954		9		15
1955		5	1	8
1956		9	4	9
1957		6	1	6
1958		8	2	12
1959		6	5	15
1960		10	2	11
1961		14	4	16
1962		11	1	8
1963		14		12
1964		12		13
1965		11		9
1966		18		15
1967		25		17
1968		19		10
1969		22		17
1970		8		10
1971		14		11
1972		12		10
1973		4		13
1974		2		8
1975		8		7
1976		13		5
1977		14		7
1978		11		5
1979		6		13

Year	M.A.	M.S.	M.B.A.	Ph.D.
1980		9		10
1981		15		9
1982		14		6
1983		16		11
1984		15		19
1985		9		9
1986		11		10
1987		13		8
1988		19		3
1989		12		12
1990		11		9
1991		7		8
1992		11		13
1993		9		5
1994		9		11
1995		5		4

Compiled in part from Dolores Nemec, "Graduates and Thesis Titles, School of Pharmacy, University of Wisconsin–Madison", F. B. Power Pharmaceutical Library, and in part from data provided by Linda Frei, School of Pharmacy graduate studies office.

Editor's Note: The data in this Appendix 4d varies in details from the data on graduate degrees included in Appendix 4a, because the two tables were developed from different sources by different compilers. Differences in the number of degrees earned (1±%), for example, might be attributable to omission of joint degrees or of degrees formerly awarded (because of administrative policy) through a department other than pharmacy.

Appendix 4e: Recipients of the Rho Chi Award, Eta Chapter

For the highest academic achievement during the freshman year.

1941— Floyd P. Hallett
1942— Robert H. Schleif
1943— August P. Lemberger
1944— Ruth Current
1945— Kermit W. Johnson
1946— Cora M. Turner,
Clarence J. Endicott
1947— Raymond E. Fiedler
1948— Richard E. Raabe
1949— Donna DeGroff
1950— Elaine Hawley
1951— Arlen E. Ward
1952— Harold A. Herman
1953— Mary K. Asperheim
1954— Elizabeth Ann Brenzel
1955— Nancy E. Lundgren
1956— Kay Iverson
1957— Vernon A. Jones
1958— John Hughes
1959— Helen A. Gilbert
1960— Robert J. Palzer
1961— Patricia Detlor
1962— Sandra Mae Carlson
1963— Judith E. Fifrick
1964— Gerald M. Cullen
1965— Patricia Kehrer
1966— Judith M. Kramer
1967— Michael Lemberger
1968— Earlene Koehler
1969— Kathleen J. Sieh
1970— Dennis A. Koranda
1971— Connie K. Kroll
1972— Randal C. Breuer
1973— Pamela A. Bongey
1974— Mary Catherine Olson
1975— Steven C. Ebert
1976— Brian C. Jensen,
Susan Marie Nordstrom
1977— Debra Ann Peterman
1978— Susan Lynn Curry,
Mary Jo Palesse
1979— Donna Paider
1980— Mark Gocker
1981— Gregory J. Teche
1982— Jon C. Schommer
1983— Arlene M. Iglar
1984— Christine L. Bergmann
1985— Andrea E. Eggert
1986— Linda Winzer
1987— See-Lun Cecilia Lau
1988— Bich Betty Ngoc Tran
1989— Karen K. Hamilton
1990— Ellen L. Peszczynski
1991— Sandra K. Killough
Michele L. Moureau
1992— Mira Suseno
1993— Michael Brown,
Marn Hong Lam,
Susan Kreul,
Jodi Volovsek
1994— Holly Franz,
Steven Brandenburg
1995— Craig Philips,
Joshua Radl

Appendix 4f: Recipients of the Lilly Achievement Award

For the senior earning the highest cumulative average during the professional years.

1966—	Patricia Williams	1982—	Elizabeth Wagner
1967—	Judith Fifrick Albers	1983—	Mary Fivizanni
1968—	Charlotte Ann Anderson	1984—	Michael Seidl
1969—	Reuben J. Adams	1985—	Jon C. Schommer
1970—	Annette L. Richter	1986—	Richard L. Berry, Jr.
1971—	Sandra L. Bartelt	1987—	Christine L. Bergmann
1972—	John H. Ruzinski	1988—	(No award given)
1973—	Kathleen J. Sieh	1989—	Gary P. Olszewski
1974—	Kent L. Hendrickson	1990—	See-Lun Cecilia Lau,
1975—	Lorna E. Goshman		Judith L. Schubert
1976—	Diane Lynn Cramer	1991—	Andrew Matulionis
1977—	Pamela Bongey	1992—	Christine L. Vogt
1978—	Cheryl Krader		
1979—	Bonnie Lou Senst	1993*—	Robert W. Kowalski
1980—	Brian C. Jensen	1994—	Staci M. Weidler
1981—	Susan Curry	1995—	Jason D. Collard

*After 1992, at the request of the donor, the award was conferred for scholastic and professional achievement, leadership, and ethical conduct (not for academic achievement alone).

Appendix 4g: Arthur H. & Margaret H. Uhl Memorial Scholarship

The scholarship has been awarded to the student entering the senior year with the highest academic achievement in coursework required by the School of Pharmacy.

1980	Susan Curry
1983	Cynthia Trobentar
1984	Sue Willborn
1985	Richard Berry
1986	Christine Bergmann
1987	Rose Cheung
1988	Gary Olszewski
1989	See-Lun Cecelia Lau and Judy Schubert
1990	Andrew Matulionis
1991	Kristine Bathke
1992	Ellen Peszczynski and Sherry Luedtke
1993	Sandra Killough
1994	Betsy Lin
1995	Mary Elliott

After the 1995–96 award, at the donor's request, the scholarship (ordinarily full resident-tuition for a year) has been given mainly on the basis of a combination of scholarship and need.

Appendix 5

Honorary Degrees and Citations Conferred by the University

FOUR GRADUATES in pharmacy have been identified from the historical records as having received an honorary degree from the University:

Frederick B. Power (London, England), LL.D., 1908

Otto J.S. Boberg (Eau Claire, Wisconsin), Pharm.M., 1925

Ko Kuei Chen (Indianapolis, Indiana), Sc.D., 1952

Oscar Rennebohm (Madison, Wisconsin), LL.D., 1962

Other recipients of an honorary doctorate who had ties to pharmacy, though to a lesser degree, were three scientists closely identified with pharmaco-industrial research and administration: Karl H. Beyer, Jr. (Sc.D., 1972), a pharmacologist; Carl Djerassi (D.Sc., 1995), a chemist; and Ralph H. Hirschmann (Sc.D., 1996), medicinal chemist.

Honorary degrees have been conferred annually, since 1856, through a highly selective all-University process that evaluates candidates from various fields of human endeavor. The second highest form of recognition is the University's honorary *citation*. Candidates from a single specialized field of endeavor are evaluated by the corresponding academic unit of the University, which proposes recipients to the Chancellor. The School of Pharmacy has drawn its candidates from two categories: (1) pharmacists in Wisconsin who have a well-established record of public service, beyond outstanding professional practice alone, and (2) persons outside the state who hold a degree from the University or have been otherwise identified closely with Wisconsin pharmacy at some stage of their career, and who have a record of outstanding achievement. Since the first pharmacy citations were awarded in 1953, recipients have been:

1953: Max N. Lemberger
Oscar Rennebohm

1954: Frederick V. Bland
Paul A. Dahl

1957: Joseph B. Burt
Jacob P. Lee
Justin L. Powers

1958: Glenn L. Jenkins
Jennings Murphy
Donald Niebuhr

1959: Frederick W. Irish
Charles O. Lee
Edwin S. Schweger

1960: Harry F. Mayer, Sr.
Sister Gladys O. Robinson

1961: Sylvester H. Dretzka
Walter W.F. Enz
Ronald J. Goggin

1962: Leo T. Gwidt
Lawrence F. Madland
Joseph V. Swintosky

1963: William J. Koch
Gordon H. Svoboda

1964: Bernard Aabel
Edward G. Farrell
Harold G. Hewitt

1965: William S. Apple
Charles F. Dahl
Lloyd M. Parks

1966: Roy A. Bowers

1967: Ole Gisvold
Lawrence J. Jones
Helger Rasmussen

1968: Paul Bjerke
Charles M. Johnson
D. Jack Myers

1969: W. Allen Daniels
Takeru Higuchi
Richard M. Hofmann

1970: Wilbur K. Baake
Sidney Riegelman
Casimir A. Zielinski

1971: Edward G. Feldman
Lyle F. Rasmussen
Arthur H. Uhl

1972: E. Richard Finger
Tom D. Rowe
Robert E. Steele

1973: Raymond Jahn
Leon Lewandowski

1974: Earl C. Hall
Edward J. Rowe
E.E. Smissman

1975: Melvin W. Green
Del A. Olszewski

1976: Eunice B. Bardell
Robert Schwartz
Dale E. Wurster

1977: Kenneth F. Finger
August P. Lemberger
Thomas D. McGregor

1978: Rodney C. Bohn
Richard G. Henry
Leslie M. Lueck, Jr.

1979: Louis W. Busse
John L. Gunsolley
Milton J. Henrichs

1980: Karl W. Marquardt
Louis B. Schroeter
Lenor B. Zeeh

1981: Roy Kuramoto
Thora M. Vervoren

1982: Joseph G. Cannon
Joseph J. Gwidt
Arthur L. McCourt

1983: Allan H. Conney
Conrad L. Sobczak

1984: Paul J. Hartung
John C. Weaver

1985: Boyd J. Poulsen
Joseph I. Sowinski

1986: Edward J. Rippie
Donald E. Van Scotter

1987: Glenn A. Sonnedecker
Hal N. Wolkoff

1988: Martin F. Stein
James E. Tingstad

1989: Armando J. Aguiar
Ronald T. Borchardt
James R. Fenno

1990: Robert W. Hammel
Mylan J. Sinclair
William A. Zellmer

1991: William L. Blockstein
Joseph A. Mollica
B. James Neuhauser

1992: Marla Ahlgrimm
Jonathan Buth
Bernard DesRoches

1993: Gary Schill
Anthony Taraszka

1994: David M. Angaran
Jordan L. Cohen
Marianne F. Ivey

1995: Norman Berndt
Norman Campbell
Joseph Gitzen

APPENDIX 6

Awards and Publications of the Faculty—A Selective List

COMPILED BY KENNETH A. CONNORS

BESIDES THESE enumerated activities and modes of recognition, numerous professional and technical activities could be cited, such as participation on the editorial boards of journals, and service as referees of manuscripts and research proposals, as reviewers of books, and as consultants to industry and governmental agencies.

I. Representative National Awards and Prizes Received

Gordon L. Amidon: Ebert Prize, 1975, 1981.

William S. Apple, Remington Honor Medal, 1967.

William L. Blockstein: Rho Chi Society Lecture Award, 1980; Remington Honor Medal, 1985.

Larry E. Boh: AACP Rufus A. Lyman Award, 1988.

Louis W. Busse: Ebert Prize, 1951; APS Advancement of Pharmacy Award, 1967.

Jens T. Carstensen: Ebert Prize, 1976; APS Pharmaceutics Award, 1977; APS Industrial Pharmaceutical Technology Award, 1979.

Kenneth A. Connors: APS Pharmaceutical Analysis (Justin L. Powers) Award, 1980.

James E. De Muth: AACP Rufus A. Lyman Award, 1993.

Melvin W. Green: Remington Honor Medal, 1976.

Robert W. Hammel: APS Economics and Administrative Science Award, 1978; Wisconsin Pharmacists Association Distinguished Service Award, 1987.

Alan L. Hanson: AACP Rufus A. Lyman Award, 1993.

Gregory Higby: AIHP Edward Kremers Award, 1995.

Takeru Higuchi: Ebert Prize, 1954; APS Physical Pharmacy Award, 1962; APS Drug Standards and Assay (Justin L. Powers) Award, 1964; APS Stimulation of Research Award, 1967; D.Sc. (h.c.) University of Michigan, 1967; Remington Honor Medal, 1983.

C. R. Hutchinson: Kitasato Medal, 1982.

Curtis A. Johnson: Paul F. Parker Award, University of Kentucky, 1994.

Edward Kremers: Ebert Prize, 1887, 1900; D.Sc. (h.c.) University of Michigan, 1913; Remington Honor Medal, 1930.

S. Morris Kupchan: Ebert Prize, 1960; APS Natural Products Award, 1965.

August P. Lemberger: UW Citation of Merit, 1977; Rho Chi Lecture Award, 1988; Higuchi Memorial Lectureship (APST, Japan), 1989; AACP, Honorary President, 1993–94; APhA Honorary President, 1996–97.

John L. Parascandola: AIHP Edward Kremers Award, 1980; George Urdang Medal, 1994.

Lloyd M. Parks: Ebert Prize, 1952; Remington Honor Medal, 1974.

David Perlman: ACS James Van Lanen Distinguished Service Award, 1977; ACS Marvin J. Johnson Research Award, 1978; Fisher Scientific Company Award, American Society for Microbiology, 1979; Charles Thom Award, Society for Industrial Microbiology, 1979.

Richard E. Peterson: Frank Blood Award, Society of Toxicology, 1993.

Daniel H. Rich: Sato International Award, Pharmaceutical Society of Japan, 1989; Vincent du Vigneaud Award, 1990; ACS Medicinal Chemistry Award, 1992; G.H. Hitchings Award, 1992; AAPS Research Achievement Award, 1992; ACS Ralph F. Hirschmann Award, 1993; Alexander von Humboldt Award, 1993; AACP Volwiler Award, 1995, Paul Ehrlich Prize, 1995.

Joseph R. Robinson: All-UW Distinguished Teaching Award, 1980; Ebert Prize, 1989; Maurice–Marie Janot Medal, 1989; Nagai Award, Japanese Pharmaceutical Association, 1990; APhA Sidney Riegelman Research Achievement Award in Pharmaceutics, 1991; D.Sc. (h.c.) Royal Danish School of Pharmacy, 1992; Founders Award, Controlled Release Society, 1993; AAPS Dale E. Wurster Distinguished Pharmaceutical Scientist Award, 1996; APhA Takeru Higuchi Research Prize for 1997.

John Scarborough: D.H.L. (h.c.) Baker University, 1993.

Charles J. Sih: Volwiler Award, American Association of Colleges of Pharmacy, 1977; Roussel Prize, 1980.

Glenn A. Sonnedecker: AIHP Edward Kremers Award, 1964; D.Sc. (h.c.) Ohio State University, 1964; Rho Chi Society Lecture Award, 1967; Schelenz Plaque, International Society for the History of Pharmacy, 1971; Remington Honor Medal, 1972; Pharm.D. (h.c.) Massachusetts College of Pharmacy, 1974; AIHP George Urdang Medal, 1976; D.Sc. (h.c.) Philadelphia College of Pharmacy & Science, 1989.

Ernst W. Stieb: AIHP Edward Kremers Award, 1967.

Bonnie L. Svarstad: APhA Research Achievement Award in Economic, Social, and Administrative Sciences, 1988.

George Urdang: Hermann Schelenz Plaque, International Society for the History of Pharmacy, 1949; Guenther Schmid Medal, 1949; J. Leon Lascoff Award, American College of Apothecaries, 1951; D.Sc. (h.c.) Philadelphia College of Pharmacy and Science, 1946.

Arthur H. Uhl: APS Stimulation of Research Award, 1965.

Peter G. Welling: D.Sc. (h.c.) University of Sydney, 1980.

Donald T. Witiak: APS Research Achievement Award in Pharmaceutical and Medicinal Chemistry, 1985.

Dale E. Wurster: APS Physical Pharmacy Award, 1965.

George Zografi: D.Sc. (h.c.) Columbia University, 1976; Ebert Prize, 1984; APS Research Achievement Award for Stimulation of Research, 1988; AAPS Dale E. Wurster Distinguished Pharmaceutical Scientist Award, 1995; AACP Volwiler Award, 1996; Rho Chi Society Lecture Award, 1997.

II. Representative Books Written or Edited*

Amidon, Gordon L.: see Connors, *Chemical Stability . . .*

Anderson, Lee; *Higby, Gregory J. The Spirit of Voluntarism: The United States Pharmacopeia, 1820–1995*, USPC, Inc., 1995.

Angaran, David, ed. *The Clinical Pharmacy Handbook*, University of Wisconsin Center for Health Sciences, Madison, 1972.

* On the scope of this list, see endnotes 30, 31 and 32 of Chapter 5 (p. 166).

Wurster, Dale E. (1947–71). Drug release from solids, protective ointments, properties of skin lipids. His most systematic work was on the percutaneous absorption of drugs, but he is probably best known as the inventor (1948) of the Wurster air-suspension coating technique. He left Wisconsin to become Dean at North Dakota State University, and later he became Dean at the University of Iowa.

Zilz, David A. (1968–96). Hospital pharmacy administration: budgets in unit dose systems, formulary development, flow chart applications, drug utilization review, expanded roles of pharmacists.

Zografi, George (1972–). His research deals with interfaces, for example the thermodynamics and time-dependent behavior of fatty acid monomolecular films, the wettability of solids, solid surface polarity, and interfacial properties of polar liquids on nonpolar phases. He maintained a research program during the five-year period when he served as Dean of the School.

These historical specifics support an important generalization: During its first century the UW School of Pharmacy pioneered graduate education and research in America, and continued to rank high among academic institutions contributing creatively to the pharmaceutical field.

Notes and References

1. *First Annual Announcement of the Department of Pharmacy of the University of Wisconsin*, Session of 1883–84, p. 5. Kremers Reference Files, F. B. Power Pharmaceutical Library, University of Wisconsin–Madison (hereinafter cited as KRF), C31(a)I, UW, 1880–1889.
2. *60th Annual Announcement, Philadelphia College of Pharmacy, 1880*. KRF, C31(a)I, Pennsylvania-Philadelphia College of Pharmacy, 1880–1889. The requirement of the thesis is also in the 1881 and 1882 announcements.
3. *Prospectus, 1883–1884, College of Pharmacy of the City of New York*. KRF, C31(a)I, New York-College of Pharmacy of the City of New York, 1880–1889.
4. *Catalogue, 1882–3, Massachusetts College of Pharmacy*. KRF, C31(a)I, Massachusetts, Mass. College of Pharmacy, 1876–1900.
5. *Contributions from the Department of Pharmacy of the University of Wisconsin*, No. 1 (Madison, Wisconsin, 1885), KRF, C31(a)I, UW, 1883–1933. This was dedicated to the Pharmaceutical Section of the Society of German Naturalists, which met at Strassburg, Germany, September 17–22, 1885.
6. *Contributions from the Department of Pharmacy of the University of Wisconsin*, No. 2, (Madison, Wisconsin, 1886), KRF, C31(a)I, UW, 1880–1889.
7. William Trelease, D.Sc., was not a student of the Department; the research reported here had been stimulated by Prof. Power.
8. F. B. Power Pharmaceutical Library, School of Pharmacy, University of Wisconsin, Madison.

9. Because of the fragmentary nature of the thesis collection, it is not easy to say when theses were *first* typed, whether they were *all* typed during these years, or how they were bound.
10. *Bulletin*, 1893–1894, School of Pharmacy. The italics, which are in the original, suggest that there may have been instances where this procedure was not followed.
11. Louis W. Busse, personal communication (October 27, 1981). Copies of the School of Pharmacy *Bulletin* for the period 1940–49 are not included in the collection of the F. B. Power Pharmaceutical Library. In 1939 the senior thesis was required, the work being taken in the form of Pharmacy 100 (Thesis), a 4-credit course offered in the fourth year of the curriculum. The compilation of graduates and thesis titles prepared by Dolores Nemec (F. B. Power Pharmaceutical Library) shows that in 1947 B.Sc. graduates presented theses, but in 1948 only a small fraction of the class wrote theses. After its elimination as a requirement, Pharmacy 100 remained available as an elective.
12. *Bulletin*, School of Pharmacy, 1893–1894, the printed announcement of the baccalaureate program first offered in 1892 (see *Proc. WPhA 1893*, 20).
13. In 1893 Kremers said, "For two years the School has offered a graduate course, but it had to wait an entire year before the first student knocked at its door." (Remarks by Kremers in *Proc. WPhA 1893*, 20). See also Ernst W. Stieb, in *Dr. Arthur H. Uhl. A Festschrift* (Madison, 1968), 35; Anon., *The Badger Pharmacist* (Madison, 1900), 180; and *Catalogue*, 1892–93, 139 and 142.
14. Schreiner held the Ph.G. (1894) from the Maryland College of Pharmacy. He earned the B.Sc. (Ph.) in 1897, the M.S. (Ph.) in 1899, and the Ph.D. in 1902. KRF, C31(a)I, Wisconsin, UW, Alumni Listing, 1886–1916.
15. Historians appear to have gotten fairly exercised about this distinction in efforts to assign priority to the first pharmaceutical Ph.D. To a scientist the distinction does not seem very important, it being a consequence solely of an administrative difficulty, which was later removed. On Kremers' complex and sometimes tense relationship with the Chemistry Department (of which he was jointly a member for more than two decades), see Aaron J. Ihde, *Chemistry as Viewed from Bascom's Hill*, [Madison, c. 1990], 279–285; 241 f.; 431; 468 f. Kremers was of course a scientist, but he was also an educator with a keen awareness of the changes he was bringing to pharmaceutical education, and, as seen in other actions, he was a man in a hurry to make those changes. He may also have wished to establish priorities, for the School and himself, for these innovations, and he therefore used, in the case of Schreiner's Ph.D., the only administrative route available to him to direct the first Ph.D. "for work in a pharmaceutical department" in the United States.
16. Figures 5.1 and 5.2 are drawn from data in Appendix 4, Table 4d.
17. Dolores Nemec, "Graduates and Thesis Titles, School of Pharmacy, University of Wisconsin–Madison", F. B. Power Pharmaceutical Library. See also D. Nemec, *Interest*, *20*, 10–31 (1981).
18. It would be possible to make a very approximate estimate of the percentage of foreign graduate students on the basis of students' names, but citizenship data are not generally available for the entire century, and the calculation would not be helpful.

Apple, William S. Prescription Pricing . . ., University of Wisconsin, Madison, 1952.

Arndt, Jack R.; Blockstein, William, eds. *Problems in Drug Abuse*, University Extension, University of Wisconsin, Madison, 1970.

Bardell, Eunice Bonow, Wisconsin Show Globe; The Wisconsin Pharmaceutical Association 1880–1980, WPhA, Madison, 1983.

Blockstein, William; Windheuser, John, eds. *Conference on Dating of Pharmaceuticals*, University of Wisconsin Extension, Madison, 1970.

Blockstein, William: see Arndt, *Problems in Drug Abuse.*

Blockstein, William; Granberg, C. Boyd, eds. *Remarkable Pharmacists*, RobLee Hill, Des Moines, 1973.

Boh, Larry E., ed. *Clinical Clerkship Manual*, Applied Therapeutics, Inc., 1992.

Carstensen, Jens T. Theory of Pharmaceutical Systems, Academic Press, New York, Vol. I, 1972; Vol. II, 1973.

Carstensen, Jens T. Pharmaceutics of Solids, Badger-Freund, Fond du Lac, Wisconsin, c. 1974.

Leeson, L.; *Carstensen, J.T.*, eds. *Dissolution Technology*, APhA, Washington, 1974. (Japanese edition, 1977).

Carstensen, Jens T. Pharmaceutics of Solids and Solid Dosage Forms, Wiley, New York, 1977.

Carstensen, Jens T. Solid Pharmaceutics: Mechanical Properties and Rate Phenomena, Academic Press, New York, 1980.

Carstensen, Jens T. Pharmaceutical Principles of Solid Dosage Forms, Technomic, Lancaster, 1993.

Carstensen, Jens T. Drug Stability, Marcel Dekker, New York, 1st edition, 1990; 2nd edition, 1995.

Carstensen, Jens T. Modeling and Data Treatment in the Pharmaceutical Sciences, Technomic, Lancaster, 1996.

Cheney, L. S.; True, Rodney. On the Flora of Madison and Vicinity . . ., University of Wisconsin, Madison, 1893?.

Christensen, Bernard. Laboratory Guide to Pharmaceutical Technique, (n.p), 1926.

Connors, Kenneth A.; Amidon, Gordon; Kennon, Lloyd. Chemical Stability of Pharmaceuticals: A Handbook for Pharmacists, Wiley, New York, 1979.

Connors, Kenneth A. Reaction Mechanisms in Organic Analytical Chemistry, Wiley, New York, 1973.

Connors, Kenneth A. A Textbook of Pharmaceutical Analysis, Wiley, New York, 1st edition, 1967; 2nd edition, 1975; 3rd edition, 1982.

Connors, Kenneth A.; Amidon, Gordon; Stella, Valentino. *Chemical Stability of Pharmaceuticals*, 2nd ed., Wiley, N.Y., 1986.

Connors, Kenneth A. Binding Constants: the Measurement of Molecular Complex Stability, Wiley-Interscience, N.Y., 1987.

Connors, Kenneth A. Chemical Kinetics: the Study of Reaction Rates in Solution, VCH, N.Y., 1990.

Hanson, Alan L. A Practical Guide to the Compounding and Dispensing of Basic Dosage Forms, 2nd ed., American Publishing Co., Madison, 1977 (3rd ed. 1982).

Higby, Gregory J., ed. *One Hundred Years of the National Formulary: a Symposium*, AIHP, 1989.

Higby, Gregory J., ed. *Pill Peddlers: Essays on the History of the Pharmaceutical Industry*, AIHP, 1990.

Higby, Gregory J. In Service to American Pharmacy: the Professional Life of William Procter, Jr., University of Alabama Press, 1992.

Higby, Gregory J., ed. *Historical Hobbies for the Pharmacist*, AIHP, 1994.

Higby, Gregory J., ed. *The History of Pharmacy: a Selected Annotated Bibliography*, Garland Publishing, 1995.

Higuchi, Takeru; Brochmann-Hanssen, Einar, eds. *Pharmaceutical Analysis*, Wiley, New York, 1961.

Kennon, Lloyd: see Connors, *Chemical Stability . . .*

Brandel, Irvin; *Kremers, Edward*. *The Balance*, Pharmaceutical Review Publishing Co., Milwaukee, 1908.

Kremers, Edward; *Urdang, George*. *History of Pharmacy . . .*, Lippincott, Philadelphia, 1st edition, 1940; 2nd edition, 1951; 3rd edition, 1963; 4th edition, 1976.

Brandel, Irvin; *Kremers, Edward*. *Percolation*, Pharmaceutical Review Publishing Co., Milwaukee, 1908.

Kremers, Edward, ed. *Pharmacopoea Augustana*, Wisconsin State Historical Society, Madison, 1927, (facsimile).

Kremers, Edward et al. *Phytochemistry*, University of Wisconsin, Madison, 3 volumes, 1931, 1933, 1934.

Kremers, Edward. trans. *The Volatile Oils* by E. Gildemeister and F. Hoffmann, Wiley, New York, 1913–22.

Mukerjee, Pasupati; Mysels, K. *Critical Micelle Concentrations of Aqueous Surfactant Systems*, United States Bureau of Standards, USGPO, Washington, 1971.

Cleland, W.; O'Leary, Marion; *Northrop, Dexter*, eds. *Isotope Effects on Enzyme-Catalyzed Reactions*: Harry Steenbock Symposium, *6th*, University Park Press, Baltimore, 1977.

Bender, George; *Parascandola, John*, eds. *American Pharmacy in the Colonial and Revolutionary Periods: A Bicentennial Symposium*, AIHP, 1977.

Bender, George; *Parascandola, John*, eds. *Symposium on Historical Hobbies for the Pharmacist*, AIHP, Madison, 1974.

Parascandola, John, ed. *The History of Antibiotics*, A Symposium, AIHP, Madison, 1980.

Whorton, James C. and *Parascandola, John*, eds., *Chemistry and Modern Society: Historical Essays in Honor of Aaron J. Ihde*, American Chemical Society, Washington, D.C., 1983.

Parks, Lloyd; Jannke, Paul; Harris, Loyd. *Inorganic Chemistry in Pharmacy*, Lippincott, Philadelphia, 1949.

Perlman, D., ed. *Advances in Applied Microbiology*, Academic Press, Vol. 17, 1974; Vol. 18, 1974; Vol. 19, 1975; Vol 26, 1980.

Perlman, D. Antibiotics, Rand McNally, Chicago, 1970.

Jones, J. Bryan; *Sih, C.*; *Perlman, D.*, eds. *Applications of Biochemical Systems in Organic Chemistry*, Wiley, New York, 1976.

Peppler, H. J.; *Perlman, D.*, eds. *Microbial Technology*, Academic Press, Vol. I, 1979; Vol. II, 1980.

Perlman, D., ed. *Vitamin B12 Coenzymes*, 1964, New York Academy of Science, *Annals*, pp. 547–921.

Hoffmann, Frederick; *Power, Frederick*. *A Manual of Chemical Analysis . . .*, Lea, Philadelphia, 1883.

Power, Frederick, trans. *The Principles of Pharmacognosy . . .*, by F. A. Fluckiger, W. Wood, New York, 1887.

Robinson, Joseph, ed. *Ophthalmic Drug Delivery Systems*, American Pharmaceutical Association, Washington, 1980.

Robinson, Joseph, ed. *Sustained and Controlled Release Drug Delivery Systems*, M. Dekker, New York, 1978.

Robinson, Joseph; Lee, V.H.L., eds. *Controlled Drug Delivery*, 2nd ed., Marcell Dekker, Inc., N.Y., 1987.

Scarborough, John, ed. *Folklore and Folk Medicines*, AIHP, Madison, 1987.

Scarborough, John. Medical Terminologies: Classical Origins, University of Oklahoma Press, 1992.

Scarborough, John. Roman Medicine, 2nd ed., University of Oklahoma Press (prob. 1997).

Scarborough, John. Drugs, Poisons, and Kings: Pharmacy and Toxicology from Attalus II of Pergamon to Cleopatra VII of Egypt, University of California Press (prob. 1997).

Sih, Charles: see Perlman, *Applications of Biochemical Systems . . .*

Sonnedecker, Glenn, rev. *Kremers and Urdang's History of Pharmacy*, Lippincott, Philadelphia, 3rd edition, 1963; 4th edition, 1976; and republished by the American Institute of the History of Pharmacy, Madison.

Hamarneh, Sami; *Sonnedecker, Glenn. A Pharmaceutical View of Abulcasis al-Zahrawi in Moorish Spain . . .*, E. J. Brill, Leiden, 1963.

Sonnedecker, Glenn; Ives, Samuel. *Pharmacy Through Four Centuries . . .*, University of Wisconsin School of Pharmacy, Madison, 1957.

Stieb, Ernst (Sonnedecker, Glenn; collab.). *Drug Adulteration: Detection and Control in Nineteenth Century Britain*, University of Wisconsin Press, Madison, 1966.

Thielke, Thomas, ed. *Drug Utilization, Monitoring and Education Parameters*, University of Wisconsin Hospitals, Madison, 1977.

True, Rodney: see Cheney, *On the Flora . . .*

Urdang, George: see Kremers, *History of Pharmacy . . .*

Urdang, George. Der Apotheker im Spiegel der Literatur, Berlin, 1921.

Urdang, George. Zur Geschichte der Metalle in den amtlichen Deutschen Arzneibüchern, Mittenwald, 1933.

Urdang, George. (with Alfred Adlung). *Grundriss der Geschichte der Deutschen Pharmazie*, Berlin, 1935.

Urdang, George. The Squibb Ancient Pharmacy, New York, 1940.

Urdang, George. The Apothecary-Chemist, Carl Wilhelm Scheele, AIHP, Madison, 1942.

Urdang, George. The London Pharmacopoeia of 1618, SHSW, Madison, 1944.

Urdang, George. Pharmacy's Part in Society, AIHP, Madison, 1946.

Urdang, George. Goethe and Pharmacy, AIHP, Madison, 1949.

Wakeman, Nellie. Guide to Chemistry 40: Plant Chemistry for Pharmacy Students, Madison, 1911.

Weinswig, Melvin. Use and Misuse of Drugs Subject to Abuse, Pegasus, New York, 1973.

Windheuser, John: see Blockstein, *Conference on Dating . . .*

Witiak, Donald T.; Newman, H.A.I.; Feller, D.R. *Clofibrate and Related Analogs*, Marcel Dekker, Inc., N.Y., 1977.

Rahman, R.G.; Witiak, Donald T. Calcium Regulation by *Calcium Antagonists*, ACS Symposium Series 201, ACS, Washington, 1982.

Witiak, Donald T.; Newman, H.A.I.; Feller, D.R., eds. *Antilipidemic Drugs: Medicinal, Chemical, and Biochemical Aspects*, Elsevier, Amsterdam, 1991.

III. Editorships of Journals

Kenneth A. Connors, *Interest* (1962–83).

Gregory J. Higby, *Pharmacy in History* (1987–)

Edward Kremers, *Pharmaceutical Archives* (1898–1903); *Pharmaceutical Review* (1901–08); *The Badger Pharmacist* (1930–41)

Joseph R. Robinson, *Journal of Parenteral Science and Technology* (formerly *Bulletin of the Parenteral Drug Association*) (1978–88)

John Scarborough, *Pharmacy in History* (1986)

Glenn Sonnedecker, *Journal of the American Pharmaceutical Association* (Prac. Pharm. Ed., 1943–48); *Pharmacy in History* (1958–63, 1985–86), *R.Ph.* (1978–79)

APPENDIX 7

Rennebohm Lectures, by Visiting Leaders in Research

1955–56 *Prof. Lyman C. Craig,* Rockefeller Institute: "Application of Extraction to Studies of Naturally Occurring Substances"; "Chemical Structure of Some Naturally Occurring Polypeptides"

1956–57 *Dr. Sidney Siggia,* General Aniline and Film Corp.: "Modern Analytical Chemistry"; "Organic Functional Group Analysis by Chemical Means"

1957–58 *Dr. Thomas J. Carney,* Eli Lilly and Company: "Major Problems in Medicinal Chemical Research"; "Natural Products in Medicinal Chemistry"

Prof. A. H. Beckett, Chelsea College of Science and Technology: "Synthetic Analgesics: Stereochemical Considerations"; "Attempts to Design Drugs Possessing a) Analgesic Activity and b) Antibacterial Activity"

1958–59 *Dr. Emil Schlittler,* CIBA Pharmaceutical Products, Inc.: "The Drug Industry and Its Research Problems"; "The Importance of Research in the Drug Industry"; "Projects for the Drug Industry"

1959–60 *Prof. Ewart A. Swinyard,* University of Utah: "Drugs: From Animals to Man"; "Experimental Seizures and Research"

1960–61 *Dr. Robert P. Fischelis,* American Pharmaceutical Association: "Pharmacy and Medical Care"; "Pharmacy and the Pharmaceutical Industry"; "Pharmacy and the Public"

1961–62 *Prof. Alfred Burger,* University of Virginia: "Medicinal Chemistry: Its Problems and Hopes"; "Nonhydrazine Inhibitors of Monoamine Oxidase"

1962–63 *Dr. Max Tishler,* Merck Sharp and Dohme Research Laboratories: "Perspectives in Pharmaceutical Chemistry"

Prof. Odin W. Anderson, University of Chicago: "The Health Service Establishment Today"

1963–64 *Prof. I. M. Kolthoff,* University of Minnesota: "The Development of Analytical Chemistry"; "Induced Reactions"

Prof. Karol Mysels, University of Southern California: "The Evolution and Properties of Thick Soap Films"; "Equilibrium Soap Films and Intermolecular Forces"

Prof. W. B. Whalley, University of London: "The Constitution of Some Nonalkaloidal Constituents of Ergot"; "The Sclerotiorin Group of Pigments: Their Chemistry and Biosynthesis"

1964–65 *Dr. Karl J. Brunings,* Geigy Chemical Corp.: "Medicinal Research: A Field of Common Interest for the Universities, Industry, and Government"; "Drugs Affecting Endogenous Amines"; "Anti-inflammatory Agents"

1965–66 *Prof. Myron L. Bender,* Northwestern University: "Organic Models of Enzymatic Catalysis"; "Mechanisms of Chymotrypsin Catalysis"

1966–67 *Prof. E. P. Abraham,* University of Oxford: "Penicillins and Cephalosporins: Their Chemistry in Relation to Biological Activity"

Dr. Karl Heusler, Woodward Research Institute, Basle, Switzerland: "Advances in Total Synthesis of ß-Lactam Antibiotics"

Prof. Klaus Hofmann, University of Pittsburgh: "The Partial Synthesis of Active Enzymes"

1967–68 *Prof. Jerrold Meinwald*, Cornell University: "Chemistry of Insect Attractants and Repellents"

1968–69 *Prof. Henry Eyring*, University of Utah: "Structure of Water and Ionic Solutions"; "Optical Rotatory Dispersion and Circular Dichroism"; "Transport Through Membranes"

1969–70 *Prof. Daniel E. Koshland*, University of California: "A Molecular Model for Enzyme Regulation"; "Peptide-Peptide Interactions"

1970–71 *Prof. James F. Danielli*, State University of New York at Buffalo: "Theory and Hypotheses in Development of Concepts of the Plasma Membrane"; "Artificial Synthesis of Living Cells"

1971–72 *Prof. Walter J. Kauzmann*, Princeton University: "Chemical and Biological Effects of Pressure: I. Fundamental Principles; II. Some Applications"

1972–73 *Dr. Julius Axelrod*, National Institutes of Health: "Regulation of the Adrenergic Neurotransmitter"; "The Use of Drugs in Biomedical Research"

1973–74 *Prof. Hans Selye*, University of Montreal: "Stress Without Distress"; "Creativity in Research"

1974–75 *Prof. Vladimir Prelog*, Swiss Federal Institute, Zurich, Switzerland: "Chirality, the Geometrical Basis of Stereochemistry"; "Boromycin, Structure and Properties"; "Chiral Concave Molecules"

1975–76 *Prof. Barnard R. Belleau*, McGill University: "Medicinal Chemistry of the Opiate Receptor: Recent Advances"; "Medicinal Chemistry of Neurotransmitter Receptors: Recent Advances"; "Translation of Recognition Effects by Active Sites: Model Studies"

1976–77 *Prof. Solomon H. Snyder*, Johns Hopkins University: "The Opiate Receptor and Its Neurotransmitter Peptides"; "Schizophrenia, Antipsychotic Drugs and the Dopamine Receptor"

1977–78 *Prof. Andrew Schally*, Tulane University: "Hypothalamic Regulation of the Pituitary Gland with Major Emphasis on Its Implications for the Control of the Productive Processes"; "Present Status of Hypothalamic Regulatory Hormones, Especially Somatostatin: Basic and Clinical Studies"

1978–79 *Dr. John R. Vane*, The Wellcome Foundation, Limited, Beckenham, England: "Prostacyclin, Platelets and Vascular Disease"

1979–80 *Dr. James Black*, The Wellcome Foundation, Beckenham, England: "Prospecting for New Drugs"; "Pharmacological Analysis of the Neurochemical Control of Gastric Secretion"

1980–81 *Prof. K. Nakanishi*, Columbia University: "Recent Studies on Visual Pigments and Bacteriorhodopsin"; "Additivity Relation in the Exciton Chirality Method; Application in Structure Determination of Oligosaccharides and Other Cases"

1981–82 *Prof. A. R. Battersby*, Cambridge University: "Biosynthesis of the Pigments of Life: Heme"; "Biosynthesis of the Pigments of Life: Vitamin B12"

1982–83 *Dr. Elwood V. Jensen*, Ludwig Institute for Cancer Research, Zürich, Switzerland: "Estrogen-receptor Interaction in Target Cells"; "Hormone Dependency of Breast Cancer"

1983–84 *Dr. Leslie L. Iversen*, Merck Sharp & Dohme Ltd.: "Neurobiology and Neuropharmacology of Alzheimer's Disease"; "Substance P and Other Brain Peptides: Basis of a New Psychopharmacology"

1984–85 *Dr. Ronald Breslow*, Columbia University: "Approaches to Artificial Enzymes"; "Imitating the Selectivity of Biochemical Reactions"

1985–86 *Dr. Max F. Perutz*, MRC Laboratory of Molecular Biology: "Protein Crystallography and New Drug Design"; "The Impact of Science on Society: Would We Be Better Off Without Research?"

1986–87 *Prof. Leroy E. Hood*, California Institute of Technology: "Immunity and the Immunoglobulin Gene Super Family"; "Biotechnology and Medicine of the Future"

1987–88 *Dr. Ira Pastan*, National Cancer Institute: "Oncotoxins: Genetically Engineered Toxins for Cancer Treatment"; "The Role of the Human Multidrug Resistance Gene in Chemotherapy"

1989–90 *Dr. Richard A. Lerner*, Research Institute of the Scripps Clinic: "Catalytic Antibodies-I"; "Catalytic Antibodies-II"

1990–91 *Prof. Phillip A. Sharp*, Massachusetts Institute of Technology: "Mechanisms of Transcription and Regulation in Eucaryotes"; "Protein-RNA Recognition in Regulation of Gene Expression"

1991–92 *Prof. Jeremy R. Knowles*, Harvard University: "An Enzymic Pericyclic Reaction: The Pursuit of Mechanism"; "Enzyme Catalysis: What Do We Understand?"

1992–93 *Prof. Carl Djerassi*, Stanford University: "The Pill at Forty-one: What Now?"

Prof. Stephen J. Benkovic, Pennsylvania State University: "How Reverse Transcriptase Transcribes"; "Catalytic Antibodies"

1994–95 *Prof. Henry R. Bourne*, University of California-San Francisco: "Diseases Tell Us How Trimeric G-Proteins Work"; "Trimeric G-Proteins: Associations with Proteins and Lipid Membranes"

1995–96 *Dr. Richard C. Mulligan*, Whitehead Institute-MIT: "The Basic Science of Gene Therapy"

Dr. Gary Nabel, University of Michigan: "Gene Therapy Strategies for Human Cancer"

Dr. James Wilson, University of Pennsylvania: "Gene Therapy: Challenges and Directions"

Dr. Jon A. Wolff, University of Wisconsin: "New Approaches to Non-Viral Gene Therapy"

Dr. Robert Debs, California Pacific Medical Center: "Cationic Liposome-Mediated Gene Transfer *in vivo* and *in vitro*"

Dr. Dorothy Nelkin, New York University: "Gene Therapy and the Public Response"

Appendix 8

The Louis W. Busse Lectures on Industrial Pharmacy

1979 *Dr. Everett N. Hiestand,* The Upjohn Company. "Material Properties That Influence Tableting"; "Time Dependent Properties in Tableting"; "Applications of Powder Flow and Compaction Theory to Tablet Machines".

1980 *Dr. K. C. Kwan,* Merck Sharp & Dohme Laboratories. "Physiological Disposition of Sulindac"; "Drug Interaction as a Pharmacokinetic Tool"; "Methods and Assumptions in Bioavailability Evaluation".

1981 *Dr. Felix Theeuwes,* Alza Corporation. "The Development of Osmotic Pumps"; "Osmotic Pumps as Rate Specified Dosage Forms".

1982 *Dr. Michael J. Pikal,* Lilly Research Laboratories. "Industrial Pharmaceutical Research: Scientific Solutions to Practical Problems"; "Heat and Mass Transfer in the Freeze Drying of Pharmaceuticals".

1984 *Dr. William R. Good,* CIBA-GEIGY Corporation. "Pharmaceutics-An Interdisciplinary Discipline"; "Transdermal Drug Delivery-Opportunities in Endocrinology"

1985 *Dr. Takeru Higuchi,* University of Kansas. "Drug Absorption Across the Skin"; "Solubility of Organic Compounds"

1986 *Dr. Francis C. Szoka, Jr.,* University of California-San Francisco. "The Role of Bilayer Contact in Membrane Destabilization: Applications to Drug Delivery from pH Sensitive Liposomes"; "The Magic Bullet Revisited—Targeting of Drugs Using Drug Carriers"

1987 *Dr. Richard E. Jones,* Genentech, Inc. "Design and Development of Protein Pharmaceuticals"; "Preformulation Characterization of Recombinant Tissue-Type Plasminogen Activator (rt-PA)"

1988 *Dr. Russell O. Potts,* Pfizer Central Research. "Stratum Corneum Lipids and Skin Barrier Function: *In Vitro* and *In Vivo* Effects"; "Can Epidermal Metabolism Affect Topical Drug Delivery?"

1989 *Dr. Felix Franks,* Pafra Ltd. "Cold Resistance in Living Organisms. What Can We Learn from Nature?"; "The In Vitro Stabilization of Proteins: Science, Engineering, Legislation and Economics"

1991 *Dr. Robert Langer,* Massachusetts Institute of Technology. "Immobilized Enzyme Bioreactors for Removal of Heparin, Bilirubin, and Cholesterol"; "Novel Polymeric Delivery Systems for Drugs and Mammalian Cells"

1991 *Dr. Elizabeth B. Vadas,* Merck-Frosst Center for Therapeutic Research. "The Development of a New Therapeutic Entity: The Search for New Therapies in Respiratory Disease"; "Formulation Development and Bioanalytical Evaluation of MK–886, an Orally Active Leukotriene Biosynthesis Inhibitor"

1993 *Dr. Lewis J. Leeson,* Ciba-Geigy Pharmaceuticals. "Generic Substitution in New Jersey—A New Jersey Drug Utilization Review Council Report"; "A Bit of Physical Pharmacy Nostaligia—The Ionization of Tetracyclines"

1994 *Dr. William J. Curatolo,* Pfizer Central Research. "Intestinal Permeability Enhancement for Poorly Permeable Drugs: Efficacy and Toxicity"; "Oral Bioavailability Improvement Strategies for Tripeptide Renin Inhibitors"

1996 *Dr. Joseph D. Andrade, Jr.,* University of Utah. "Direct Reading Biosensors: Analytical Chemistry without Instruments"; "Scientists and the Public Understanding of Science"

Index

"I" after a page number means that entry refers to an Illustration. "n" after a page number is followed by the number of endnote or footnote to which it refers (e.g., 137n8). Abbreviations in the index are identified, for the most part, in the table "Common Abbrevations" on page 11.

A

B

C

F

G

H

M

N

O

P

R

S

T

U

V

W

Y Z

Library of Congress Cataloging-in-Publication Data

The University of Wisconsin, School of Pharmacy : its first century /
by Carl Buckner ... [et al.].
p. cm.
Includes bibliographical references and index.
1. University of Wisconsin—Madison. School of Pharmacy—History. 2. Pharmacy colleges—Wisconsin—Madison—History. I. Buckner, Carl, 1941– .
[DNLM: 1. University of Wisconsin—Madison. School of Pharmacy. 2. Schools, Pharmacy—history—Wisconsin. QV 19 U57 1997]
RS111.W6U55 1997
615'.1'071177583—dc21
DNLM/DLC 97-20473
for Library of Congress CIP